Taking the Guesswork Out of Adopting
a Plant-Based Lifestyle

By Tracey Eakin

This book is dedicated to my husband, Larry, and our children, John and Noah, for all of their love and support.

Cover picture by David M. Bowers, www.dmbowers.com.

Table of Contents

This book was created for the busy individual who does not have time to read a lengthy, in-depth book, or the substantial amount of scientific evidence which demonstrates the immense health benefits of eating a low-fat, whole food, plant-based lifestyle, but nonetheless wants to improve their health by incorporating positive change into their already hectic schedule.

For this very reason, this book is not designed to go in great detail into the sound, scientific foundation for these recommendations. However, I have included all of my sources and a vast amount of additional information that can be accessed through the multitude of Internet sites referenced in the text. Think of this book as the "Cliff Notes version" of the most comprehensive, scientifically-based nutrition information available today from those in the forefront of nutrition research and lifestyle medicine.

I wish you the very best of health.

Diseases/Disorders Impacted by Our Food Choices

Heart Disease (hypertension, elevated cholesterol, elevated triglycerides, angina)

Atherosclerosis (depending upon the arteries affected, can result in strokes, dementia, macular degeneration, hearing loss, periodontitis, aortic aneurysm, heart attacks, bowel infarction, kidney failure, back pain, degenerative disk disease, ruptured lumbar disks, impotence, intermittent claudication, and gangrene)

Type II Diabetes

Overweight/Obesity

Gastrointestinal Diseases (bad breath, gastro esophageal reflux disease (GERD), hiatus hernia, ulcers, gastritis, leaky gut (increased intestinal permeability), fatty liver disease, chronic viral hepatitis, gallstones, gallbladder disease, appendicitis, diverticular disease, irritable bowel syndrome, ulcerative colitis, Crohn's disease, colon polyps, diarrhea, constipation, enterohepatic circulation, hemorrhoids)

Autoimmune Disorders (type I diabetes, rheumatoid arthritis, juvenile rheumatoid arthritis, inflammatory arthritis, psoriatic arthritis, systemic lupus, lupus erythematosus, lupus nephritis, multiple sclerosis, ulcerative colitis, Crohn's disease, fibromyalgia, scleroderma, myasthenia gravis, ankylosing spondylitis, relapsing polychondritis, Hashimoto's thyroiditis, glomerulonephritis, nephrotic syndrome, idiopathic thrombocytopenic purpura, vitiligo)

Cancer

Osteoporosis

Arthritis

Kidney Stones and Kidney Disease

Recurrent Urinary Tract Infections

Gout

Varicose Veins

Acne

Depression

Dementia/Alzheimer's Disease

Headaches

Asthma

Sexual Dysfunction

Infertility

Autism

Children's Bed Wetting

Insomnia

Sleep Apnea

Frequency and Intensity of Colds, Viruses, and Allergies

How a Plant-Based Lifestyle Can Help to Prevent, Arrest, Reverse, or More Effectively Battle Chronic, Degenerative Diseases

Conventional medicine in Western civilization approaches chronic, degenerative diseases by treating their symptoms with pharmaceutical drugs and surgical interventions, not by addressing the causes of these diseases. This often results in a temporary fix but ongoing progression of the underlying condition.

Furthermore, improving our biomarkers of health (blood pressure, cholesterol, triglycerides, blood sugar, etc.) via prescription medications can provide us with a false sense of security. These are not diseases themselves but indicators of disease. Per Drs. Alona Pulde and Matthew Lederman, treating the symptoms without addressing

> *"Every time you eat or drink you are either feeding disease or fighting it!"*
> *Eat Healthy and Thrive*

the underlying disease is like disabling the "check engine" light on our car and thinking we've fixed the engine! They provide the example that significantly lowering the elevated blood pressure of a man through medications will still leave him with a 20% greater chance of a cardiac event than a person who mediates their high blood pressure with healthy lifestyle choices because the medicated man's arteries remain sick.

As Denis Burkitt, MD described, "If a floor is flooded as a result of a dripping tap, it is of little use to mop up the floor unless the tap is turned off. The water from the tap represents the cost of disease, and the flooded floor represents the diseases filling our hospital beds. Medical students learn far more about methods of floor mopping than about turning off taps, and doctors who are specialists in mops and brushes can earn infinitely more money than those dedicated to shutting off taps." In addition, the drug companies are more than happy to sell rolls of paper towels so patients can buy a new roll every day for the rest of their lives.

Prescription drug and surgical intervention also carry associated risks and negative side effects. Switching to a low-fat, whole food, plant-based lifestyle does not increase any health risks and the only side effects are good ones like increased energy, sustained weight loss, and fewer aches and pains. That doesn't mean that prescription drugs and surgical intervention are never appropriate. It just shouldn't be our first line of defense unless it is an emergent situation. We need to fully educate ourselves on the risks and rewards of the proposed initiatives from objective sources that don't stand to make money on the selection of the protocol. That being said, I'm also not suggesting that you totally disregard the recommendations of your medical professional. I am suggesting that you listen to their suggestions but also seek out answers of your own. I highly recommend that you visit some of my Must See Web Sites listed at the following link: http://www.traceyeakin.com/articles.html. These sources provide some of the research to which I am referring.

Lifestyle medicine complements conventional medicine. It seeks to resolve the root cause for the symptoms by incorporating better lifestyle choices.

Our bodies have a tremendous ability to heal if given the right circumstances and our bodies never cease trying to heal as long as we are alive. Surprisingly, genetics is not the overriding factor which determines whether or not we suffer with a chronic, degenerative disease(s). The food and drink that we put into our bodies is the single most powerful factor that determines our health and well-being. They are the greatest contact that we have with our external environment, so we need to make every bite and sip count.

Inherited traits are passed from one generation to another by way of genes. Some genes act as dictators, such as those that determine eye color, hair color, or blood type. Other genes act as advisors. They make suggestions. An example of this kind of gene may be a person's resistance to diseases. In this case, a person's environment, their lifestyle, helps to determine if the gene is expressed. Per T. Colin Campbell, PhD, Jacob Gould Schurman Professor Emeritus of Nutritional Biochemistry at Cornell University, "Genes do not determine disease on their own. Genes function only by being activated, or expressed, and nutrition plays a critical role in determining which genes, good or bad, are expressed." Matthew Lederman, MD puts it this way, "Genetics loads the gun, but environment pulls the trigger." Neal Barnard, MD explains that "Genes are not the only thing we pass down from generation to generation. We also pass down recipes." A major review on diet's impact on cancer, prepared for the U.S. Congress in 1981, estimated that genetics only determines about 2-3% of total cancer risk. Even the most powerful breast cancer-associated genes, BRCA1 and BRCA2, have an estimated penetrance of anywhere from 30-70%, and that is the chance of developing the disease by age 70, not dying from it, and these estimates tend to come from women with both genes and a strong family history of the disease, which means the actual gene penetrance is even lower for women without family histories. There is an entirely new field emerging to study the factors influencing the expression of genes. It is called epigenetics and it studies methylation, or how sections of our genetic code are turned on and off.

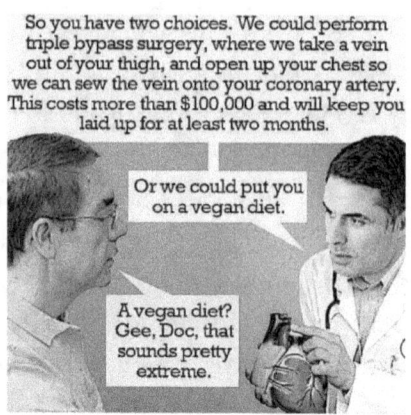

Vascular Disease

High-fat, high-cholesterol diets encourage atherosclerosis in our arteries. When the arterial lining becomes damaged by cigarette smoke combustion, oxidized cholesterol, and cow's milk protein antibodies, then fat and cholesterol can deposit underneath the lining, and form plaques. The subsequent narrowing of the arteries from these plaques can result in elevated blood pressure. Just think of what happens to the water pressure in a hose if you cover up half of the opening with your thumb.

Cholesterol only exists in foods with an animal origin. There is no dietary need to consume cholesterol as our bodies make all that we need. A high-fat diet can encourage our bodies to make too much cholesterol. Cholesterol is basically the same in all animals. Switching from red meat to white meat will not likely reduce our cholesterol levels. 35% of heart attacks occur in people with a cholesterol level between 150 and 199. Per Caldwell B. Esselstyn, Jr., MD, those with cholesterol levels below 150, without the assistance of medication, are essentially heart-attack proof. Cholesterol levels below 150 are attainable with a low-fat, plant-based lifestyle.

Only 10% of heart attacks are the result of the blockages that are the target of surgical intervention such as bypass surgery, angioplasty, and stents. These blockages have developed slowly over time and whereas they may cause angina, they are much more stable and have likely developed collaterals, tiny vascular threads that bypass the blockage to provide blood downstream. It is the more volatile, juvenile plaques that are more likely to rupture. Our bodies respond by clotting the rupture, which can result in a blockage.

Caldwell B. Esselstyn, Jr., MD of the Cleveland Clinic and Dean Ornish, MD have demonstrated that heart disease need not be the number one killer of Americans. A low-fat, plant-based lifestyle can not only halt the progression of the disease, but has the ability to reverse the damage as well.

Here are a few comments from thought leaders in this field:

- "Do not confuse the absence of symptoms with the absence of disease. Heart attacks and strokes can strike without warning. 40% of the time, the first symptom of vascular disease is instant death." Pam Popper, ND
- "Stroke attacks with no warning signs, and results in death 25% of the time." Rip Esselstyn
- "If you have vascular disease anywhere, you have it everywhere." Terry Mason, MD
- "Heart disease is a choice." Michael Greger, MD

Type II Diabetes

Carbohydrates and sugar are not the cause of type II diabetes. Excess intramyocellular lipids, excess fat within our muscle cells, paralyze insulin activity. When food is digested, starches are broken down into glucose, the body's preferred source of fuel. The glucose permeates the gut barrier and circulates in the bloodstream. The hormone insulin is released at this time to unlock the doors to our cells so that glucose can enter and be burned as energy in our cell furnaces, the mitochondria. Excess intramyocellular lipids can act as gum stuck in each cell's door lock. Insulin, the key, is unable to open the door to our cells and as a result, glucose builds up in our bloodstream and spills into our urine. A person can be slender and still have excess lipids within their muscle cells. A low-fat, plant-based lifestyle will enable the excess lipids to dissipate and insulin can regain its sensitivity, sometimes in as little as a week. *Make sure to notify your doctor of your planned diet change as the subsequent improvement in your insulin sensitivity will likely dictate a decrease in your medication. Do not adjust any medication without the knowledge and consent of your doctor.*

Overweight/Obesity

Obesity can be a gateway condition to a host of chronic, degenerative diseases including heart disease, type II diabetes, osteoarthritis, and some types of cancer.

The most comprehensive study of nutrition ever conducted, The China Study, demonstrated that not all calories are created equal when it comes to weight loss and long-term weight maintenance. This finding has shattered the calories in/calories out theory as those following a plant-based lifestyle generally weigh less than those that eat the standard American diet, yet consume more calories. The China Study found when they compared similarly active plant-based Chinese to Americans eating the standard American diet, the average caloric intake of the Chinese was 30% higher, yet their average body weight was 20% lower. This may be explained by the way our bodies process the macronutrients of protein, carbohydrate, and fat:

Our bodies do not store protein. Once our protein needs are met, any excess is excreted through our kidneys. The typical protein-excessive

American diet can harm the kidneys. "In healthy people with no apparent diseases, it is estimated that they lose about 1/3 of their kidney function by the time they reach the age of 70 because of the high protein nature of the rich, American diet." John McDougall, MD

Carbohydrates are used to fuel the body. Excess carbohydrates are first stored as two pounds of glycogen in the liver and muscle tissues to be used when fuel is scarce. Any excess after that is burned off as body heat in a process known as thermogenesis.

Fat is stored easily and relatively unchanged on the body. Our bodies needed this ability to survive as a species when food was scarce. This is not necessarily an advantage in developed nations in today's world where food loaded and layered with added fat, sugar, and salt is too easily accessible.

Adopting a low-fat, plant-based lifestyle enables us to eat when we are hungry, to eat until we are satisfied but not stuffed, and still attain and maintain an optimal weight. This way of eating is nutrient dense but calorie dilute so that the food we consume fills us up before the calories fill us out! The nutrient dilute, calorie dense standard American diet has produced a malnourished, overweight nation. A plant-based lifestyle does not require the counting of calories, fat grams, protein, grams, etc., but as a general guideline, T. Colin Campbell, PhD recommends that we aim for 80% carbohydrate, 10% protein, and 10% fat.

We can't out exercise a bad diet, so with your physician's blessing, incorporate more activity into your day to complement your new way of eating, rather than to attempt to offset the consumption of unhealthy foods.

Gastrointestinal Diseases

We have the most contact with the external environment via our gastrointestinal tract. The food and drink we consume has a direct impact on our digestive system. Animal products contain high levels of sulfur-containing amino acids like methionine and cysteine. They are also disproportionately high in Omega 6 fatty acids. Therefore, an animal-based diet is very acidic, very irritating, and pro-inflammatory. A low-fat, plant-based lifestyle contains an appropriate amount of sulfur-containing essential amino acids and the proper balance of Omega 3 and Omega 6 essential fatty acids, which has an alkaline and anti-inflammatory effect on our blood and body tissues.

Autoimmune Disorders

A special note to those adopting this lifestyle to try to halt an autoimmune reaction: please be patient. It can take longer to arrest an autoimmune disorder than it does to begin to see progress with other chronic, degenerative diseases.

A leaky gut (increased intestinal permeability) is thought to be the mechanism by which partially digested animal proteins (peptides), especially dairy proteins, gain inappropriate access to the bloodstream, causing the immune system to react by making antibodies against what it recognizes as foreign material. If these circulating antibodies locate amino acid sequences identical to the peptides for which they were created, they can attack these identical sequences, even if they are a normal part of the human body. Dietary fat, cholesterol, chronic NSAID pain reliever use, and other toxins can damage this sensitive gastrointestinal layer. It can take up to four months to heal a leaky gut once the repeated injury to this intestinal barrier has ceased.

A plant-based lifestyle can halt the progression of an autoimmune disorder, but the damage already incurred cannot be reversed.

Cancer

Per Michael Greger, MD, diet (food and alcohol) is the number one cause of cancer. Only 5-10% of cancer is in our genes, in our family history.

Food influences the hormones that fuel cancer growth. Hormones encourage growth, not just in normal body tissue, but in cancer tissue as well. That is why the main goal of many cancer drugs is to block estrogen's activity. The more fat that exists in a person's diet, the more bile acids the liver creates in order to digest that fat. When the bile acids reach the intestine, they are converted into sex hormones by the bacteria present in the intestine, further elevating hormone levels. The vast majority of plant foods are naturally low in fat. Those that are higher in fat are truly healthy fat. Minimizing artificially extracted added oils helps to minimize excess hormone production and keeps our immune system running strong. In fact, vegetable oils are the strongest promoter of cancer with which we commonly come into contact. When the percentage of fat calories in the diet exceeds 15%, cancer incidence increases. Animal-based food is generally 20%-70% fat. Plant foods are generally less than 10% fat. The more body fat a woman has, the more estrogen she makes, because fat stores act like estrogen factories. Both men and women that have more body fat tend to have less sex hormone-binding globulin (SHBG) in their blood. SHBG's job is to bind with excess hormones and render them inactive and unable to promote cancer. Your percentage of calories from fat should not exceed 15%.

Fiber encourages the efficient elimination of waste products, hormones, carcinogens, and excess medications by binding with and neutralizing the waste material and carrying it out of the body in a timely manner with the bowel movement. If inadequate fiber exists in the diet and hormones waiting to be excreted sit in the intestine for longer than they should, they could be re-absorbed into the bloodstream and re-circulate, further elevating your hormone levels. This is called enterohepatic circulation. Fiber is only found in plant foods.

Phytates have a wide-range of health-promoting properties including anti-cancer activity. Foods high in phytates include beans, grains, nuts, and seeds. Phytates affect all of the principal pathways of malignancy. Phytates are antioxidant, anti-inflammatory, immune enhancing, detoxing, influence cell differentiation (the reversion of cancer cells back to the behavior of normal cells), encourage anti-angiogenesis (not just preventing the formation of new blood supplies to tumors but also disrupting existing supply lines), and augment natural killer cell and neutrophil (our first line of defense) activity. Phytates have also been found to inhibit the metastatic process by inhibiting human colon and breast cancer cells from producing tumor invasion enzymes. Phytates help patients to experience fewer symptoms from the chemotherapy and help to prevent the normal drop in immune cells and platelets, all without any bad side effects. Dietary phytate might be the most important variable governing the frequency of colon cancer. Phytate is a powerful inhibitor of the iron-mediated production of hydroxyl radicals, a particularly dangerous type of free radical. So the standard American diet may be a double whammy, the heme iron in muscle meat plus the lack of phytate in refined plant foods to extinguish those iron radicals.

Per Neal Barnard, MD, research indicates that if a dietary change is to alter the course of this disease, the changes need to be significant.

Additional information regarding cancer, such as the following questions, can be found in the chapter Commonly Asked Questions:

- Does sugar feed cancer cells?

- Is soy safe to eat if I have cancer or if I'm a cancer survivor? Is soy safe for boys and men?
- Are there any additional strategies I can implement if I want to try to prevent cancer, if I have cancer, or if I'm a cancer survivor?

Dairy

Humans are the only species to drink the milk of another species and we are the only species to drink milk passed the age of weaning. Milks differ from species to species in order to accommodate each newborn's specific needs. Buying organic milk will eliminate the growth hormones and antibiotics injected into the cows, but will not eliminate the naturally occurring bovine hormones found in cow's milk that are designed to grow a 60-pound calf into a 600-pound cow in 6 months.

Consuming dairy products has been shown to increase the level of insulin-like growth factor 1 (IGF-1) in the bloodstream. IGF-1 is a powerful stimulus for cancer cell growth.

The most comprehensive study of nutrition ever conducted, The China Study, determined that according to traditional regulatory criteria, casein, which comprises 87% of cow's milk protein, is the most significant carcinogen ever discovered. Drinking 2% or skim milk, or consuming other low-fat dairy products, will reduce the amount of fat you are consuming but will actually increase the proportion of casein.

Due to modern farming practices, cows are milked throughout their pregnancies, which can result in 33 times the normal level of estrogen in milk produced from cows in the later stages of their pregnancies compared to cows that are not pregnant. To minimize cancer risk, it is critical that circulating hormone levels be minimized.

For a comprehensive analysis of the dangers of dairy, please refer to the article entitled The Dangers of Dairy located on my website on the following page: http://www.traceyeakin.com/articles.html.

Cancer feeds on cholesterol. It uses it to create the estrogen that helps it to thrive and is required for the "lipid rafts in its plasma membranes" that are important not only for tumor survival, but also for tumor migration and invasion. Eliminating cholesterol-laden animal products and consuming plant phytosterols such as sunflower and pumpkin seeds and soybeans, naturally help to eliminate cholesterol. Statins do not have the same effect as phytosterols, in fact, the long-term use of cholesterol-lowering statin drugs is associated with more than double the risk of both types of breast cancer: invasive ductal carcinoma and invasive lobular carcinoma.

When meat is cooked, heterocyclic amines form in the muscle tissue. Heterocyclic amines are carcinogenic. The longer the meat is cooked and the hotter it gets, the more heterocyclic amines form. Grilled chicken is the largest source of heterocyclic amines in the US diet. When meat is grilled, it also forms polycyclic aromatic hydrocarbons on the surface of the meat. These substances are carcinogenic as well.

Many human cancers, including leukemia and some tumors of the colon, breast, ovary, prostate, and skin, have absolute methionine dependency. They need methionine to survive. Chicken and fish are particularly rich sources of methionine, although it is also found in high concentrations in all animal products. Methionine restriction is best achieved with a plant-based lifestyle.

Cancer may use a molecule found in animal products, Neu5GC, to trick our immune system into feeding it with inflammation. Our bodies still recognize cancer tumors as "self". When the tumor incorporates Neu5Gc into itself, our bodies do not recognize the Neu5Gc as "self", and incite a low-grade inflammation that ultimately feeds the cancer tumor.

Meat is void of fiber and protective phytochemicals.

For a comprehensive analysis of the dangers of chicken and fish, please refer to the articles on my web site at:

http://www.traceyeakin.com/articles.html:

- Is Switching from Beef to Chicken Really Improving Our Health?
- Fish...Is It Good for Us?

Osteoporosis

Osteoporosis is not a result of inadequate calcium intake. It is the result of overly rapid calcium loss. Countries with the highest dairy consumption also have the highest incidences of osteoporosis.

Our bodies must maintain a slightly alkaline pH in our blood and body tissues in order to accommodate all of the chemical reactions that take place on an ongoing basis. Meat and dairy products are high in the sulfur-containing amino acids, methionine and cysteine, which when digested, create a very acidic environment. Our bodies must access material from our primary buffering system, our bones, in order to neutralize the acid and restore balance. This can result in an ongoing draw on bone material which can lead to osteoporosis. Studies have found that no level of calcium supplementation can keep a person in positive calcium balance (keeping more calcium than we are losing) as long as a person eats the rich, American diet. It is like trying to keep a bathtub full of water by turning on the faucet but not putting a plug in the drain. This excess passage of calcium through the kidneys also provides the raw material for 95% of kidney stones.

Dietary sodium, caffeine, alcohol, and smoking have also been found to accelerate the passage of calcium and other material from our bones.

Weight-bearing exercises are important as they rebuild lost bone density. Adequate sunlight for vitamin D, and fruits and vegetables for vitamin C, potassium, magnesium, and boron, are also important for bone health. Look to plant sources for calcium such as green, leafy vegetables, legumes, figs, and sweet potatoes.

Vitamin D helps us to absorb calcium and is very protective against cancer. It must undergo molecular changes in the kidneys and the liver before it can be activated. When we consume dairy products, the huge load of calcium it provides signals to our bodies not to activate the vitamin D as that could cause our bodies to absorb too much calcium, which could be toxic. Those with the highest dairy consumption have been found to have the lowest levels of activated vitamin D.

Contact Me

For questions and/or assistance with the transition to a low-fat, plant-based lifestyle, don't hesitate to contact me at traceyeakin@gmail.com or 724.469.0693. My web site is www.traceyeakin.com/. Please subscribe on my web site to my free, monthly e-newsletters. You can unsubscribe at any time.

As a Plant-Based Nutrition Counselor, I provide clients with a summary of the findings from medical doctors and PhD's in the forefront of nutrition research and lifestyle medicine. It is not intended to replace competent medical advice. Notify your physician before making any significant lifestyle change, such as the transition to a plant-based lifestyle, as the subsequent improvement in your health may decrease your need for certain medications. This is critically important to diabetics on medication, especially insulin, those on high blood pressure medication, and those with compromised kidney function. It is imperative that you do not alter your medication regimen or stop it entirely without the advice of your physician. Your physician is welcome to contact me with any questions.

What is a Plant-Based Lifestyle?

Before we go any further, I think it is worthwhile to review two commonly used descriptions for this way of eating: plant-based and vegan. They are similar but not completely inter-changeable, however, there are times throughout this book where it is simply easier to use the word vegan. Plant-based is the abbreviated way of referring to a low-fat, whole food, minimally processed, plant-based lifestyle. It emulates what the best scientific studies have demonstrated as the optimal way for our species to eat. It refers solely to an eating style and is described in detail below.

Vegan is a philosophy for living life and is more inclusive than just what a person eats. It is an ardent belief that all sentient beings have bodily integrity and the inviolate right not to be exploited, that all sentient beings have their own innate self worth and exist for their own sake. For these reasons, they have the right not to be killed for food, to make clothing, to be experimented on, or to exploited as entertainment for humans. Therefore, vegans do not eat any foods of animal origin; they don't wear leather, wool, or silk; they don't buy personal care and household products that have been tested on animals or contain animal products; and they don't frequent circuses, Sea World, zoos, or petting zoos. Food manufacturers often label foods without animal products as vegan, indicating that the food *may be* an acceptable option for you. Please keep in my however, that not all vegan food is health promoting, and this book will help you to discern if it is. Twizzlers and Oreos are vegan, but they certainly are not what you would eat to be healthy.

The Four Food Groups

Just enjoy a variety of minimally processed whole grains, legumes (beans, peas, and lentils), vegetables, and fruit, with raw, unsalted nuts and seeds and minimal added oils. Eat when you are hungry and until you are satisfied but not stuffed, and you will be providing yourself with the best chance of a long and healthy life. The closer foods are to their natural state, that is the less processed and/or refined that they are, the better. This way of eating will provide you with all of the vitamins, minerals, essential amino acids that comprise protein, essential fatty acids, fiber, antioxidants, and other phytochemicals that you need to lead a vibrant, healthy life. It is simply the best way to nourish loved ones of any age from infants after weaning (for detailed information on introducing new plant-based foods to weaning infants, Pregnancy, Children, and the Vegan Diet by Michael Klaper, MD and Vegan for Life by Jack Norris, RD and Virginia Messina, MPH, RD are wonderful resources) to the elderly to elite athletes.

Another way to look at this lifestyle is, at each meal, fill half of your plate with starch (oats, groats, whole grains, whole wheat, buckwheat, wheat berries, bulgur, farro, brown rice, wild rice, barley, rye, sorghum, triticale, corn, quinoa, millet, beans, lima beans, peas, lentils, potatoes, sweet potatoes, yams, winter squash, pasta, whole grain and sprouted grain breads, cous cous, gnocchi, etc.). Fill the other half with one or two non-starchy vegetables and fruit.

Try to start all meals with a piece of fruit, soup, a salad, or steamed/braised vegetables. This enables you to begin filling your stomach, and expanding the stretch receptors in your stomach, with nutrient-dense, but calorie-dilute plant foods. Following this with starches finishes filling your stomach with nutrient-dense, but also more calorie-dense plant foods.

It is easy to meet the recommended intake of short-chain omega 3 essential fatty acids, alpha-linolenic acid, with a plant-based lifestyle.

The daily recommendation for women is 1.1 grams which can be met by adding 1 tablespoon of ground flax seed or 3 walnut halves. The daily recommendation for men is 1.6 grams which can be met by adding 1 1/3 tablespoons of ground flax seed or 4 walnut halves.

Supplement with vitamin B_{12}. For more information on supplements, see my chapter on supplements.

Doctors have found the most success transitioning patients to a low-fat, plant-based lifestyle with the implementation of a 21-day immersion program, that is, giving it 100% for just 21 days. It provides the maximum results in a short, defined time period. It facilitates a rapid change in tastes to lighter fare. It also coincides with findings that it takes about 21 days to change a habit. This is the recommended approach. Give it all you've got for three weeks and see how good you can feel and how much your health can improve in such a short amount of time. Then keep your attention short-term and focus on subsequent three-week increments.

If a gradual approach is more your style, then begin by changing as much as you feel you can. While any change toward a healthier lifestyle is beneficial, please continue your progress by making additional changes every 21 days and understand that the results will be more subtle and may take longer to achieve.

Studies have shown that in order to arrest and reverse vascular disease, halt an autoimmune disorder, or alter the course of cancer, dietary changes must be significant. When battling these diseases, in addition to the elimination of all animal products, added vegetables oils should also be eliminated or at least scrupulously minimized.

No matter which method you decide is best for you to transition, please be patient with yourself. You've likely eaten the standard American diet all of your life and it will take an investment of time up front to form healthy, new habits. If at any point you feel that this lifestyle is just not for you, please take some time to think about what is working and what is not before you abandon all of your efforts. You may be surprised that with a little tweaking of one or two aspects, you can be back on the road to success. There is a wonderful online, plant-based community and almost unlimited resources to tap. People that have probably faced and surmounted the very obstacle(s) in your way can be very helpful getting you over it too.

When making any lifestyle change, take time to plan how the change will be implemented and maintained so that you are less likely to revert to your old ways in a crisis. Consider beginning on a Saturday or Sunday when you will have more time and flexibility than a busy Monday morning. Look ahead three weeks and make sure there are no major disruptions planned, such as a vacation or business trip, that might make your initial transition more difficult than it needs to be. This is a great article on successfully incorporating lifestyle changes. I highly recommend you read it and give it a try :

http://www.huffingtonpost.com/2012/11/26/life-changes-how-to-create-habits_n_1970105.html#es_share_ended.

There is no calorie, fat gram, or protein gram tracking. *Just eat a wide and colorful variety of minimally processed whole grains, legumes, vegetables, and fruit, with raw, unsalted nuts and seeds and minimal added oils, until you are satisfied, but not stuffed. Remember to avoid all animal products (beef, chicken, turkey, pork, fish, shellfish, dairy, eggs, casein, whey, and gelatin) and minimize added oils.*

If after you begin your test drive, you feel hungry, deprived, or lethargic, ask yourself these questions:

Are you eating enough?

It is sometimes difficult to imagine that you will lose weight and regain your health without the deprivation that accompanies fad diets, however, now you are working in harmony with your body, not against it, and your weight and wellness will begin to reflect that. As long as you eat when you are hungry and stop when you are satisfied, but not stuffed, you should begin to see positive results. A number of biological safety mechanisms will begin to kick in if you do not give yourself enough to eat. It signals to your body that a famine has set in and in response, your body will slow your metabolism in an attempt to preserve every calorie possible. It will also encourage you to binge. You may hold out for a while, but eventually, you will succumb. The drive to survive that has kept our species alive is just too strong for you not to give in at some point.

If you are a quantitative person that thrives with numbers and guidelines and enjoys tracking statistics about what you are eating, then remember the Rule of 10. As a minimum, make sure to eat 10 calories for each pound of your ideal weight to prevent your metabolism from screeching to a halt. For example, if your ideal weight is 130 pounds, then you should make sure you are eating at least 1,300 calories per day. You will very likely continue to lose weight even if you are eating more than this minimum.

Are you eating enough starch?

Starch is your body's preferred primary source of fuel. It is also provides the most satiety (satisfaction, fullness) out of all of the food groups, with potatoes topping the list. You should not feel hungry, deprived, or lethargic if you are giving yourself enough of the right foods to eat. Green and yellow vegetables are extremely healthy, but if they are comprising too large a proportion of your meals, you are likely going to remain hungry and feel as though you are lacking energy. Try incorporating more starch (oats, groats, whole grains, whole wheat, buckwheat, wheat berries, bulgur, farro, brown rice, wild rice, barley, rye, sorghum, triticale, corn, quinoa, millet, beans, lima beans, peas, lentils, potatoes, sweet potatoes, yams, winter squash, pasta, whole grain and sprouted grain breads, cous cous, gnocchi, etc.).

Guidelines for an Incredible Plant-Based Journey:

- Eat when you are hungry and stop when you are full but not stuffed.
- When building your meals, starch takes center stage on your plate (oats, groats, whole grains, whole wheat, buckwheat, wheat berries, bulgur, farro, brown rice, wild rice, barley, rye, sorghum, triticale, corn, quinoa, millet, beans, lima beans, peas, lentils, potatoes, sweet potatoes, yams, winter squash, pasta, whole grain and sprouted grain breads, cous cous, gnocchi, etc.) accompanied by one or two vegetables, and fruit. Raw nuts and seeds can accent meals.
- Incorporate 1 tablespoon of ground flax seed or 1 tablespoon of walnuts each day for Omega 3 essential fatty acids.
- Enjoy 1 ounce of raw, unsalted nuts each day, unless you are allergic to them and/or have not yet reached your optimum weight.
- Supplement with vitamin B_{12}, preferably in the form of methylcobalamin.
- Eat your food in as close to its natural packaging as possible (the least processed/refined).
- Omit all animal products (beef, chicken, turkey, pork, fish, shellfish, dairy, eggs, casein, whey, and gelatin).
- Omit or minimize added oils. There is plenty of naturally occurring fat in the plant kingdom.
- Adequately hydrate with filtered water.
- Get adequate, but not excessive sunshine: 10-15 minutes between 10 am and 2 pm without sunscreen on at least your face, neck, and arms in the spring, summer, and fall. This should provide you with adequate vitamin D stores during the winter.
- Get adequate but not excessive, recuperative sleep.
- With your doctor's blessing, incorporate regular exercise.
- It takes 3 weeks to change a habit and our taste buds. Keep your focus short-term on 3-week increments.

Meal Ideas

Most people have about nine favorite dinners that they frequently prepare. The Cancer Project's 3-3-3 plan is simple. Find three meals that you already love that do not contain any animal products or added fat. Add to them three more meals that you already love that can easily be adapted by removing or substituting the animal products and by removing or significantly decreasing the amount of added oils (spaghetti with marinara sauce instead of meat sauce; bean burritos instead of beef burritos; steamed mixed vegetables over brown rice instead of chicken with mixed vegetables over rice). Then select three new recipes that you'd like to try and you'll have a new set of nine recipes to enjoy.

The recipes for these meal ideas are found later in the book.

Here are some delicious and simple ideas for breakfast. You may find that you stay satisfied longer if you include a natural source of plant protein:

- one pound (before cooking) non-starchy vegetables followed by anything listed below. For an explanation of this strategy, please refer to my chapter entitled Suggestions for Maximizing Weight Loss and the section that reads: *Incorporate a larger proportion of non-starchy vegetables into your day, but not so many that you are left feeling hungry or deprived.*
- *FAST!* – old fashioned oatmeal cooked with filtered water or non-dairy milk with any or all of the following ingredients:
    - fresh, frozen, or dried fruit
    - 100% fruit spread
    - cinnamon
    - pure vanilla extract
    - nuts and/or seeds
    - semi-sweet, non-dairy, chocolate chips
    - 1 tablespoon chia seed, hemp seed, or ground flax seed
    - wheat germ

- *FAST!* - The Ultimate Smoothie (page 107)
- *FAST!* - Michael Greger, MD's Smoothie (page 108)
- *FAST!* - It's Easy Being Green Smoothie (page 109)
- *FAST!* - Michael Greger, MD's Pumpkin Pie Smoothie (page 110)
- whole grain pancakes (if you are using a mix, make sure it doesn't contain any animal products) made with water or non-dairy milk (no need to add eggs)
- Spelt-Blueberry Pancakes (page 111)
- Tofu French Toast (page 112)
- *FAST!* - whole grain frozen waffles
- Apple-Maple Fusion Topping (a wonderful way to extend your pure maple syrup) (page 113)
- Healthy Hash Brown Casserole (page 114)
- home fries, braised mixed vegetables, toast, and fruit (page 115)
- gRAWnola using Date Paste (page 116)
- Better-Than-Boxed Strawberry and Oat Breakfast Cereal (page 117)
- *FAST!* - Nabisco Shredded Wheat and Bran, Post Grape-Nuts, Bob's Red Mill Natural Granola (which doesn't contain any added fat), or Post Lightly Sweetened Spoon-Sized Shredded Wheat cereal with non-dairy milk and a side of fresh fruit
- *FAST!* - fresh fruit, non-dairy yogurt, and whole grain toast or Ezekiel English muffin topped with 100% fruit spread
- Maple-Cinnamon Peanut Butter Toast (page 120)
- *FAST!* - Latin American breakfast (whole grain toast topped with rinsed, drained, and heated black beans, salsa, and Dijon mustard)
- *FAST!* - canned garbanzo beans, rinsed and drained
- Scrambled Tofu (page 121)
- Vegan Blueberry Muffins with Crumb Topping (page 122)
- Spring Fling Scones (page 124)
- Quick Rice Pudding (page 267)

The following recipes can be used either for lunch or dinner, or even as snacks. Make extra of favorite recipes to freeze or for lunch or dinner the following day:

Salads:
- Fruit and Vegetable Salad (page 129)
- Hot Skillet Salad (page 130)
- Potato Salad (page 131)
- Couscous Confetti Salad (page 132)
- Three Bean Salad (page 133)
- Corn and Black Bean Salad (page 134)
- Mexican Corn Salad (page 135)
- Hoppin' John Salad (page 136)
- Marinated Lentil Salad (page 137)
- French Lentil Salad (page 138)
- Marinated Zucchini and Chickpea Salad (page 139)

Soups and Stews:
- *FAST!* - Dr. McDougall's soup cups
- *FAST!* - Progresso 99% Fat Free Lentil soup
- *FAST!* - Amy's Organic Low Fat Split Pea Soup
- *FAST!* - Thai Kitchen Instant Rice Noodle Soup (Garlic & Vegetable and Spring Onion only), these are a healthier version of Oodles of Noodles
- *FAST!* - Black Bean and Salsa Soup (page 141)
- *FAST!* – touch your lightly steamed asparagus with an immersion blender and add a little sea salt for a delicious, refreshing soup
- *FAST!* – a delicious pea soup can be made by cooking peas, Earth Balance buttery spread, sugar, salt, apple juice or water, non-dairy milk, and tomato juice
- Summer Minestrone (page 142)
- Red Bean, Potato, and Arugula Soup (page 144)
- Cabbage Soup (page 145)
- Carrot and Red Pepper Soup (page 146)
- Zuppa Vegana: Italian, Bean, and Kale Soup (page 147)

- Lifting Lemon-Garlic Rice and Lentil Soup (page 148)
- Quick and Easy Potato Soup (page 151)
- Leek, Spinach, and Potato Soup (page 152)
- Mexican Corn Chowder (page 153)
- *FAST!* - Speedy International Stew (page 155)
- Peruvian Quinoa Stew (page 156)
- Curried Potato Stew (page 158)
- Kapusta (page 159)

Sandwiches, Burgers, and Quesadillas:

- *FAST!* - whole grain tortilla wrap stuffed with your choice of non-fat refried beans, corn, brown rice, low-fat guacamole, romaine lettuce, tomato, salsa, non-dairy sour cream, hot sauce, and black olives (or skip the tortilla and place everything in a big bowl over a generous bed of romaine lettuce)
- *FAST!* - whole grain tortilla wrap stuffed with your choice of hummus (homemade or store bought, purchasing the one with the lowest fat), low-fat guacamole, romaine lettuce, tomato, and black olives
- *FAST!* - whole grain tortilla stuffed with black bean dip, peppers, tomatoes, and romaine lettuce
- *FAST!* - vegetable wraps made by rolling diced vegetables, avocado slices, olives, sunflower seeds, and anything else you can think of rolled in collard green leaves or romaine lettuce leaves
- 3-2-1 Hummus (page 161)
- Eggless Salad Sandwiches (page 162)
- "Chicken" Salad Sandwich (page 163)
- Savory Sandwiches (page 164)
- Mock Tuna Salad (page 165)
- Italian eggplant sub (baked eggplant slices, pizza sauce, and mushrooms on a multi-grain sub roll)
- veggie burger (without soy protein isolate), baked sweet potato or sweet potato fries, and steamed vegetables
- Colleen's Chickpea Burgers with Tahini Sauce (page 166)
- BBQ Peanut Sweet Potato Burgers (page 167)

- *FAST!* - meatless Sloppy Joes, baked French fries, and steamed vegetable (page 169)
- *FAST!* – cheeseless quesadilla made with hummus instead of cheese to hold all the vegetables in place

Pizza:

- *FAST!* - Tofurky brand frozen pizzas, available at most grocery and health food stores (although enjoy only occasionally as it is high in fat)
- homemade pizza with homemade or store bought whole wheat pizza crust, or Boboli whole wheat shell, pizza sauce, Daiya shredded mozzarella cheese (although go easy on this because it is still high in fat and is highly processed), vegetarian pepperoni (go easy on this too as it is highly processed), and your choice of favorite vegetable toppings.

Casseroles:

- An easy casserole can be made by steaming jasmine rice and fresh vegetables using tomato juice or other liquid.
- *FAST!* - No Fuss Casserole (page 172)
- Potato and Veggie Casserole (page 173)
- Red Bean Casserole (page 174)
- Asparagus and Chickpea Casserole (page 175)
- Creamy Vegan Broccoli and Rice Casserole (page 176)
- Cheezy Casserole (page 177)

Other Entrees and Side Dishes:

- *FAST!* - Serve Progresso 99% Fat Free Lentil soup over steamed brown rice or mashed potatoes
- *FAST!* - sweet potato, vegetarian baked beans, asparagus, and watermelon
- *FAST!* - Near East toasted pine nut cous cous, canned three bean salad, steamed broccoli, apple and clementine wedges, Aurora Cranberry Health Mix, and Michael Greger, MD's recipe for hibiscus lemon water
- *FAST!* - Southern Stir-Fry (page 180)

- baked potato bar (topped with pepper, nutritional yeast, steamed vegetables, soup/stew, meatless chili, salsa, black beans, corn, corn and black bean salad, pico de gallo, low-fat guacamole, or fat-free salad dressing)
- mashed potatoes (made with the potato skins still on and blended with an unsweetened, non-dairy milk), corn, peas, and a plant-based brown gravy
- Parsnip Mashed Potatoes (page 181)
- Mashed NOtatoes (page 182)
- Tex Mex Potatoes with Tofu Taco Topping (page 183)
- black bean and sweet potato burrito with corn and tomatoes
- Sweet Potato and Blue Corn Enchiladas (page 185)
- pasta (whole wheat is preferable) or gnocchi with a meatless/cheeseless sauce, and Italian Mushrooms (page 186)
- Spaghetti with Zucchini and Lemon (page 187)
- Raw Vegan Pesto with Zucchini Noodles (page 188)
- Zucchini "Noodles" with Sesame-Peanut Sauce (page 189)
- pasta ribbons (eggless noodles), vegetarian baked beans, steamed spinach, and fresh strawberries
- Halusky (page 190)
- steamed, mixed vegetables with Hunan or Szechuan sauce over brown rice
- Easy Thai Noodles (page 191)
- Hurry-Up Hoisin Tofu and Vegetables with Rice Noodles (page 192)
- Sichuan Tofu with Garlic Sauce (page 193)
- Chef AJ's Fiesta Rice (brown rice, black beans, corn, peas, shredded zucchini, shredded carrots, red onion, and 1 cup of pico de gallo)
- Near East Whole Grain Blends Brown Rice Pilaf or Wheat Pilaf or Near East Toasted Pine Nut Couscous, any variety of bean mixed with your favorite salsa and onions that have been sautéed in water, and a steamed vegetable
- Black Beans and Rice Extravaganza! (page 194)
- Rice Medley (page 195)
- North African Couscous Paella (page 196)

- Sweet Roasted Corn Risotto (page 197)
- Rainbow Risotto (page 199)
- Easy Vegan Greens and Beans with Sassy's Seedalicious Topping (page 200 and 201)
- Super Vegetarian Chili served over mashed potatoes (page 202)
- Hearty Chili Mac (page 203)
- Greek-Style Cannellini and Vegetables (page 205)
- Beans Florentine (page 207)
- *FAST!* - Disorderly Lentils (page 208)
- Savory Miso + Spiced Lentil Power Plate (page 209)
- Skillet-Popped Lentils, Harvest Skillet Style (page 212)
- Spiced Lentils and Rice (page 214)
- Mary McCartney's Hot Pot Recipe (page 215)
- Menestra (page 216)
- Roasted Ratatouille (page 218)
- Vegan Macaroni and Cheese (page 219)
- Chipotle Mac and "Cheese" with Roasted Brussels Sprouts (page 220)
- Cheesy Cauliflower Sauce (page 221)
- Cheezy Sauce (page 222)
- No-Meat Loaf, homemade mashed potatoes, mushroom gravy, and steamed broccoli (page 223)
- Polenta with Black Beans and Mango Salsa (page 225)
- Tofu Nuggets (page 226)
- Spicy Kale (page 227)
- Braised Mixed Vegetables (page 228)
- Simple Bean and Vegetable Braise (page 229)
- Sure Fire Roasted Vegetables (page 230)
- Easy Roasted Beets (page 232)
- Try making spinach by cooking it in white wine, garlic, kosher salt, and pepper.

Special Holiday Recipes:

- Thanksgiving Day Special: Bread and Herb Casserole (page 234)
- Vegan Green Bean Casserole (page 236)
- Yam and Apple Casserole (page 237)
- New Year's Day Special: mashed potatoes, sauerkraut, and green beans (page 238)

Pressure Cooker Recipes:

- Mushroom Chili (page 240)

Salad Dressings:

- *FAST!* - Splash your salad with some seasoned rice vinegar or the juice from a freshly squeezed orange.
- *FAST!* - Whisk together until smooth 1 tablespoon tahini, 1 teaspoon agave nectar, a dash of salt, and enough water to achieve the desired consistency.
- Low-Fat Tahini-Chickpea Dressing (page 242)
- Artichoke Brazil Nut Dressing (page 243)
- Hidden Cashew Ranch Dressing (page 244)

Snacks/Desserts:

Snacks and desserts do not have to be taboo. If they are done correctly, they can help you to bridge the gap between meals so that you don't arrive at the table, or go to bed, ravenously hungry. Keep in mind though that snacks and desserts are not meals. They should be smaller than meals and be strategically placed throughout your day to help you avoid feeling deprived. Ideally, they should be packed with nutrition just like your breakfast, lunch, and dinner. Keep some healthy snacks with you when you are on the run so that you never feel compelled to sacrifice nutrition because you lack access to healthy food. Everything you eat and drink should add to your health, not detract from it.

- *FAST!* - Microwave small red potatoes and store in the refrigerator for a fast snack/meal on the go. Eat plain just as you would an apple. You'll be surprised how good they taste!
- *FAST!* - canned garbanzo beans, rinsed and drained (You can even buy single-serve, pull-top cans to eat on-the-go!)
- *FAST!* - vegetables or whole wheat pita bread dipped in low-fat hummus
- *FAST!* - McDougall soup cup
- *FAST!* - Edward & Sons Brown Rice Snaps (unsalted plain, onion garlic, and tamari sesame flavors) or Wasa crisp bread alone or topped with hummus
- *FAST!* - chopped vegetables dipped in fat-free salad dressing or a salad dressing with fat derived from whole plant sources such as the tahini (ground sesame seeds) in goddess dressing.
- *FAST!* - apple slices dipped in natural, unsalted and unsweetened peanut butter (be careful not to overdo as peanut butter is high in fat)
- *FAST!* - a handful of raw nuts or seeds (be careful not to overdo as they are high in fat), for those who like more precise estimates, one ounce, or about 16 almonds, 22 peanuts, 11 walnut halves, 25 pistachios, or 16 cashews
- *FAST!* - a handful of trail mix
- *FAST!* - Popcorn (popcorn kernels either air-popped or microwaved in a lunch-sized brown paper bag) topped with a dash of cayenne pepper or spritzed with Bragg's Liquid Aminos and apple cider vinegar, then topped with chlorella and nutritional yeast. *Commercial microwave popcorn bags are sprayed with a carcinogenic chemical to keep the popcorn from sticking to the sides of the bag. Microwave popcorn also contains the World War I chemical warfare agent and poisonous gas, phosgene, that can cause bronchiolitis obliterans, a generally irreversible, fatal lung condition, and the artificial butter flavoring diacetyl, which can*

cause another potentially fatal disease referred to as "popcorn lung".

- *FAST!* - baked chips/tortillas with fat-free bean dip or salsa
- *FAST!* - whole grain pretzels
- Broccoli and Peanut Dip (page 246)
- "Ranch" Dip (page 247)
- Roasted Chickpeas with Red Chili Pepper Flakes (page 248)
- microwave potato chips (page 249)
- *FAST!* - fresh fruit
- *FAST!* - a handful of dried fruit (be careful not to overdo and make sure they do not contain added sugar or sulphites, as sulphites have been implicated as an asthmatic enhancer)
- *FAST!* - 100% frozen fruit bars
- *FAST!* - non-dairy yogurt mixed with fresh or frozen fruit and frozen ahead of time in plastic popsicle forms
- *FAST!* - non-dairy yogurt mixed with cocoa; it's a great night-time snack when you are craving chocolate!
- *FAST!* - sorbet (make sure it doesn't contain any dairy)
- *FAST!* - Larabars, Go Raw bars, or Kashi bars (make sure it doesn't contain any dairy or soy protein isolate)
- *FAST!* - whole grain fruit Newton cookies
- *FAST!* - Newman-O's cookies (enjoy only occasionally as they are highly processed and higher in fat)
- *FAST!* - Tofutti non-dairy ice cream, chocolate fudge treats, and Cuties ice cream sandwiches (enjoy only occasionally as they are highly processed and higher in fat)
- Oatmeal Goji Berry Balls (page 250)
- Energy Balls (page 251)
- Chewy, Homemade Granola Bars (page 252)
- Apple Cranberry Crisp (page 254)
- Oatmeal Banana Bites (page 255)
- Banana-Maple Oatmeal Cookies (page 256)
- Adonis Cake (page 258)
- Vegan Double-Layer Pumpkin Cheesecake (page 260)
- Raw Carrot Cake with Vanilla Cream Frosting (page 261)
- Mocha Mousse (page 263)

- Chocolate Raspberry Mousse (page 264)
- Chocolate Cherry Nirvana Smoothie (page 265)
- Nicer Krispie Squares (page 266)
- Quick Rice Pudding (page 267)

Beverages:

Water is the only essential beverage past weaning. Due to the pervasiveness of pollution on our planet, water should be filtered. Aim for 64 ounces a day.

Try taking it up a notch by adding fresh lemon to your water. According to professional Ironman triathlete, Brendan Brazier, lemon may add the following benefits (http://myvega.com/blog/2012/top-5-reasons-drink-lemon-water):

- Support immune function-lemons are high in the antioxidant vitamin C, demonstrate anti-inflammatory effects, and increase iron absorption; the saponins in lemons also display antimicrobial properties
- Alkalize the body
- Aid digestion via citrus flavonols; vitamin C is also believed to reduce the risk of peptic ulcers caused by Helicobacter pylori
- Clear skin-believed to purge toxins from the blood by stimulating the liver, thereby helping to keep skin clear of blemishes; vitamin C and other antioxidants help to combat free radical damage which can lead to wrinkles; can be applied directly to skin to reduce the appearance of scars and age spots
- Promote healing

Willing to take it one step further? According to Michael Greger, MD, the following recipe may produce the highest antioxidant beverage in the world (http://nutritionfacts.org/video/better-than-green-tea/):

8 cups (0.5 gallon) of filtered water

4 bags of any tea in which hibiscus is the first ingredient (or you can blend 4 teaspoons of organic dried hibiscus flowers that have been soaked overnight in just enough water to cover them)

juice of 1 lemon

3 tablespoons of erythritol or you can blend in some dates (optional)

½" fresh ginger root (optional)

1 teaspoon amla powder (optional)

handful of fresh mint leaves (optional)

Combine and cold brew in the refrigerator overnight. In the morning, remove the tea bags (I just keep the tea bags in the container.), shake it up, and drink it. For a bonus, blend 1 cup on high with a bunch of fresh mint leaves and/or fresh or frozen berries.

Two cautionary notes with regard to hibiscus:

Per Dr. Greger, hibiscus tea is sour and therefore potentially erosive to the enamel on our teeth, so make sure not to brush your teeth immediately after consumption. Instead, we should swish some water around in our mouth to wash some of the acid off of our teeth. Drinking it through a straw would also minimize exposure.

Manganese is an essential trace mineral, a vital component of some of our most important antioxidant enzymes. Hibiscus tea contains an impressive quantity of manganese. If we consume too much from regular tea, our bodies limit absorption and increase excretion. Because of this, there is little evidence that dietary manganese poses a risk with regular tea. There is, however, no evidence available for hibiscus tea specifically, and using hibiscus leaves instead of hibiscus tea further increases the available amount of manganese. So to be on the safe side when consuming hibiscus tea, Dr. Greger recommends no more than about 1 quart per day for adults and ½ quart per day for children.

Another suggestion from Michael Greger, MD, albeit a little simpler than the recipe above, is to dissolve matcha in filtered water and enjoy. Matcha is powdered green tea leaves. According to Dr. Greger, matcha provides whopping loads of nutrition and maximizes the phytonutrient absorption in tea. I found matcha in my local health food store.

Commercially prepared 100% cranberry juice only has 50% of the whole berry's phytonutrient power due to its processing. Dr. Greger developed his own whole food cranberry juice recipe:

2 cups filtered water

handful of frozen cranberries

8 teaspoons of erythritol

fresh ginger root (optional)

Blend in a Vitamix blender. A less powerful blender may not be up to the task. For a tasty variation, replace the frozen cranberries with frozen dark cherries, the juice of a whole lemon, and some fresh mint leaves.

Refer to the Vitamix chapter to find out how you can get a discount on the shipping expense of your Vitamix order.

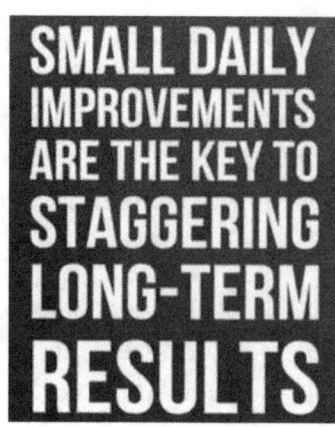

SMALL DAILY IMPROVEMENTS ARE THE KEY TO STAGGERING LONG-TERM RESULTS

Suggestions for Maximizing Weight Loss

Our bodies continually strive to maintain homeostasis, or balance. Initially, our bodies may fight us in our quest to reach our optimum weight, in a misguided effort to maintain this balance. Be patient, it may take a couple of weeks before you start to see the results on the scale, but your body will eventually get the message and start cooperating.

Adopting a low-fat, plant-based lifestyle is a safe and healthy way to reach and maintain your optimal weight. The weight loss should be gradual but steady. It is possible, however, to reach a plateau from time to time. Fine tuning what you are eating will more than likely kick your weight loss back into gear. Consider incorporating these additional suggestions and watch for the positive effect on your bathroom scale:

Be stringent about fat.

Do not include added oils, even if they are of vegetable origin. This includes plant-based buttery spreads and imitation cheese.

Avoid high-fat plant foods such as nuts, nut butters, seeds, olives, avocado, coconut, and full-fat tofu. Ground flax seed and walnuts are excellent sources of Omega 3 essential fatty acids, however, our bodies do not require that much. One tablespoon of ground flax seed or walnuts is all that needs to be incorporated into our daily food choices.

Prepared hummus can vary widely in fat content depending upon how much tahini is used and if vegetable oils are added.

Chef AJ suggests substituting beans for nuts in recipes.

It may take a little extra effort at clean-up time, but avoid coating cookware and bake ware with oil. According to Caldwell Esselstyn, MD, even a quick squirt of vegetable oil spray can result in one tablespoon of added oil!

When eating out, don't hesitate to ask your server to go light on the oil. Sometimes, I think chefs that are not as familiar with plant-based meals feel as though they have to replace the meat and dairy they leave out with something else, like oil, in an effort to keep the dish tasty. This is simply not the case.

We only need about 5% of our calories to come from fat, or about 10 grams per day, and that is easily obtained naturally from the plant kingdom. Limit fat to 2-3 grams per serving and/or less than 10% of calories from fat.

Incorporate a larger proportion of non-starchy vegetables into your day, but not so many that you are left feeling hungry or deprived. Studies have shown that, on average, we tend to eat the same *weight* of food each day. If we replace calorically dense food with calorically dilute food, we should lower our overall caloric intake without feeling deprived. Chef AJ starts each day with one pound of something green. Throughout the day, she eats another pound of cooked, green vegetables. This does not include the salads and fruits that she eats daily as well. I follow Chef AJ's suggestion and have found that consuming two pounds of non-starchy vegetables each day is not only easily attainable once it becomes a habit, but is also enjoyable, and it really helps to temper my appetite throughout the day. On the days when I have gone without this quantity of non-starchy vegetables, I feel ravenous all day long and my appetite seems to be unquenchable.

Now if you've gotten over the initial shock of my recommendation to eat a pound of non-starchy vegetables as the first part of your breakfast, let me assure you that it is possible to incorporate this into your lifestyle, and it's a good idea even if you aren't trying to lose weight. I've never met with a client that admitted not eating enough vegetables. We all think we eat enough, at least I did until I began incorporating one to two pounds a day. I highly recommend a mix of non-starchy vegetables, such as a stir-fry mix. Not only does this increase the variety of vegetables eaten, it also makes eating a pound in one sitting much more enjoyable. Sometimes, I'll cook a pound of green beans when I'm looking for a change in the morning. I follow this with a smaller portion of what I would normally eat for breakfast so that I am sustained until lunch. This portion size, which measures just under 3 cups, is not outside the realm of possibility and you can work up to it gradually.

Avoid highly processed whole grains such as bread, bagels, tortillas, pasta, dry cereal, pretzels, crackers, and other flour products. These foods are digested and absorbed differently than whole foods. Replace instead with oats, groats, whole grains, whole wheat, buckwheat, wheat berries, bulgur, farro, brown rice, wild rice, barley, rye, sorghum, triticale, corn, quinoa, millet, beans, lima beans, peas, lentils, potatoes, sweet potatoes, yams, and winter squash.

Don't drink your meals. Liquid calories provide less satiety than solid food containing the same amount of calories.

Avoid the dense calories of dried fruit. Opt for fresh or frozen fruit instead.

Limit fresh fruit to one piece per day. Fructose, the sugar found in fruit and processed foods, is the only form of sugar that can be converted to fat by the body under normal circumstances.

Make sure you are listening to your body's satiety cues. Years of yo-yo dieting and the subsequent binging that ultimately results can damage your finely tuned instinct of knowing when you've had enough to eat. Pay close attention to your feeling of fullness so that you don't overeat. If you are unsure if you are full, stop eating for ten minutes, then reassess.

According to Jeff Novick, MS, RD, LD, LN, if you have to exercise more than 150 minutes per week in order to lose or maintain your weight, then you are simply eating too many calories.

A principle called volumetrics can be applied to plant-based food as well to help you maximize your weight loss. The rule is simple. Just look at the food's nutrition label. If one serving has fewer calories than grams of weight for that one serving, it is a good choice to eat as the weight of the food will fill you up before the calories of the food fill you out!

If you are trying to lose weight, aim for a weight loss of about one pound per week. Adjust your intake accordingly. If you have a lot of weight to lose to attain your ideal weight, an overly rapid rate of loss could put you at a higher than average risk for gallstones.

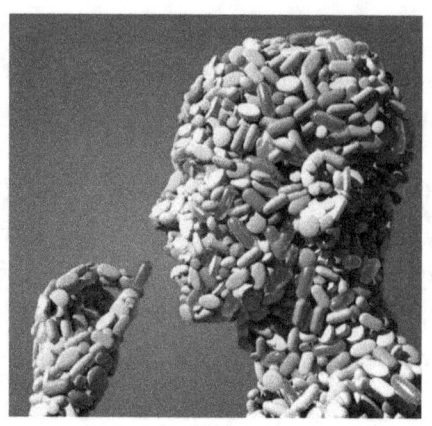

Supplements

The best way to obtain vitamins, minerals, protein, essential fatty acids, antioxidants, and other phytonutrients is in their natural packages. In other words, in whole plant foods as nature created them. A low-fat, plant-based lifestyle, which incorporates a moderate variety of whole plant foods, should provide everything we need to lead a vibrant life, with the exception of vitamin B_{12} and vitamin D.

Vitamin B_{12}

Vitamin B_{12} is actually created by micro-organisms. Before we thoroughly washed our fresh fruits and vegetables, we consumed adequate amounts of this vitamin because it was created by the micro-organisms that lived in the soil that was left on our produce. People who consume meat and dairy products obtain their vitamin B_{12} from the animals and animal products that they are consuming; the animals obtained their vitamin B_{12} from consuming dirt as they were eating off of the ground.

Now do I think we should stop washing our produce and keep eating animals? No. The cons of doing so far outweigh any pros and supplementation is simple.

There are actually four main forms of vitamin B_{12}: cyanocobalamin, hydroxocobalamin, methylcobalamin, and adenosylcobalamin. The most common form of vitamin B_{12} is cyanocobalamin. However, it contains a molecule of cyanide which makes it a more stable form of the vitamin. The vast majority of people will not experience adverse effects but those with compromised kidney function may not detoxify cyanide as well as those with full functioning kidneys. Even if you and your family have fully functioning kidneys, why introduce cyanide into your bodies if you don't have to? To be safe, a hydroxocobalamin and/or methylcobalamin form is recommended but may be harder to find. Hydroxocobalamin is the form of the vitamin usually found in food and the form usually administered by an injection from your doctor.

I recommend Pure Vegan Methylcobalamin B_{12} 500 mcg Spray. It is available through Amazon. It is a great tasting spray which works well for children and adults that don't like to swallow pills.

The recommended daily dose is just 5 mcg daily although the absorption rate is lower for an oral dose. If the smallest dose you can find is about 500 mcg, then one dose once a week should be more than adequate. There is no known harm in exceeding the recommended daily dose.

If you feel that you are already deficient in vitamin B_{12}, which can occur if someone follows an entirely plant-based lifestyle for more than three years without supplementation, then the following protocol is recommended by Jeff Novick, MS, RD, LD, LN:

2,000 mcg daily for two weeks, then reduce to about 10-100 mcgs once a day or 1,000 mcgs twice a week.

Vitamin D

Vitamin D is actually a hormone that assists your body with calcium absorption. It has also been found to be protective against cancer. It is naturally acquired by the action of sunlight, specifically UVB rays, on our skin, converting cholesterol into vitamin D. Adequate sun exposure during the spring, summer, and fall is efficiently stored in your body fat and will provide the reserves that you need through the winter when sun exposure is limited.

Matthew Lederman, MD of Exsalus Health & Wellness Center in Los Angeles, California, takes the guess work out of adequate and safe sun exposure. He created the following table to assist people in determining how much sun is appropriate given their skin type and local climate. You can locate the daily UV Index (UVI) for your zip code at http://www.weather.com/.

Skin Type	UVI: 0-2	UVI: 3-5	UVI:6-7	UVI: 8-10 & Tanning	UVI: 11+
Always Burn & Never Tan	None	10-15 min.	5-10 min.	2-8 min.	1-5 min.
Easily Burn & Rarely Tan	None	15-20 min.	10-15 min.	5-8 min.	2-8 min.
Occas. Burn & Slowly Tan	None	20-30 min.	15-20 min.	10-15 min.	5-10 min.
Rarely Burn & Rapidly Tan	None	30-40 min.	20-30 min.	15-20 min.	10-15 min.
Never Burn & Always Dark	None	40-60 min.	30-40 min.	20-30 min.	15-20 min.

This chart is shared with permission from Matthew Lederman, MD (www.transitiontohealth.com/) and the Center for Nutrition Studies online certificate program (www.nutritionstudies.org).

The research doesn't support any further artificial supplementation, especially if a deficiency has not been determined. If a deficiency is diagnosed, then the first course of action should be to obtain the deficient nutrient(s) from whole plant food sources of that nutrient or from natural sunlight in the case of vitamin D, then recheck your deficiency at an interval recommended by your physician.

Matthew Lederman, MD has conducted extensive research into the development of supplement recommendations and the supposed benefits that they convey. He found the research to be inadequate and poorly substantiated.

In addition, as more credible research is conducted, the more examples researchers are finding where artificial supplementation causes nutrient imbalances and in some cases actually increases mortality.

So eat a diverse variety of whole grains, legumes, vegetables, and fruits, with some nuts and seeds, minimally processed with no/minimal added oil, supplement with vitamin B_{12}, and get adequate but not excessive sun exposure, and you can be on your way to a more vibrant life.

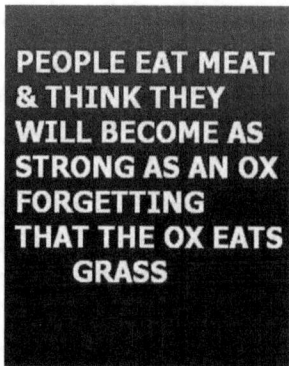

PEOPLE EAT MEAT
& THINK THEY
WILL BECOME AS
STRONG AS AN OX
FORGETTING
THAT THE OX EATS
GRASS

Meat and Dairy Substitutes

The meat and dairy substitutes have improved IMMENSELY since I first began eliminating animal products in 1988. For the vast majority of the products I recommend below, I truly feel they taste comparable or even better than what they are replacing. To save you a lot of time and money trying all of the different brands available, here are my best recommendations. Feel free to try other brands if you do not prefer any of those listed below:

In general, anywhere you used to put meat, you can put beans instead. Here are a few examples:

- Substitute black beans in Mexican dishes.
- Substitute kidney and pinto beans in soups as they seem to hold their shape despite prolonged cooking.
- Garbanzo beans develop a creamy texture after blending that resembles sour cream or cheese in dips. Try adding dried cherries and chipotle (smoked hot chili pepper) for an incredible taste!

Milk

Non-dairy milks are a perfect substitute for dairy-based milks and can be used in all instances just like milk. Almond, coconut, and soy milk, which are available unsweetened, plain, or flavored, are available in grocery stores. Unsweetened almond milk most closely resembles my memories of cow's milk. I would recommend unsweetened almond milk for use in preparing mashed potatoes and other dishes where a sweet taste would not complement the dish. I would recommend using coconut milk when preparing desserts and other sweet dishes.

Butter

Earth Balance Whipped Organic Natural Buttery Spread is available in most grocery stores. It can be used as a spread, to fry, to sauté, and to bake. It is free of hydrogenated oils and has zero grams of trans fat. It also does not contain any genetically modified organisms (non-GMO). It is however, a processed, added fat and as such, should be used sparingly.

Cheese

Daiya is available as slices, as shreds, and in blocks, and can be found in most grocery stores. It tastes so good that many plant-based food manufacturers have begun to use Daiya in their products, such as vegan frozen pizzas and macaroni and cheese. Until recently, there have not been any suitable cheese substitutes. Veggie Slices came very close in taste, but in order for the cheese to melt when heated, casein was used as an ingredient. The most comprehensive study on nutrition to-date, The China Study, found casein to be the most significant carcinogen ever discovered. So avoid any cheese substitutes that contain casein. The shredded Daiya does not taste good right out of the bag, but melted, it tastes very good. Be careful however, as Daiya is higher in fat so treat yourself only occasionally. You may find it difficult to completely break away from cheese when you continue to eat foods, even 100% plant-based foods, that have a taste, texture, and appearance of the real thing. If you find this to be the case, avoid cheese substitutes entirely, and give yourself three weeks to adjust to their absence. Your tastes and habits will change and you will wonder why you were ever so hooked on cheese in the first place. All that will be left will be fond memories!

Nutritional yeast, not brewer's yeast, may be sprinkled on top of pasta and mixed into recipes for a cheesy flavor. Nutritional yeast can be found in most health food stores.

Yogurt

Coconut and soy milk yogurt are very good substitutes for dairy-based yogurt and can be found in most grocery stores. I did not care for almond milk yogurt or non-dairy Greek yogurt. I've never tried dairy-based Greek yogurt so it may just be that I wouldn't like it either. If you can't find the non-dairy yogurt that you are looking for in your local grocery store, try your local health food store.

Coffee Creamer

Soy and coconut creamer, both regular and flavored, are available in most grocery stores. It is an acquired taste for most, so I highly recommend that if you prefer not to drink your coffee black, give yourself one pint to get used to it. Once you do, you'll never want to go back to half-and-half!

Mayonnaise

Follow Your Heart Original Vegenaise Dressing & Sandwich Spread is available in most grocery stores. It is a very close substitute to mayonnaise. It is high in fat, so make sure to use it sparingly.

Cream Cheese

Tofutti Better Than Cream Cheese doesn't taste exactly like cream cheese, but when you sprinkle some of your favorite Mrs. Dash on top, it tastes a lot better and does have the texture of real cream cheese. This is a highly processed product, so use sparingly.

Sour Cream

Tofutti Sour Supreme Better Than Sour Cream doesn't taste exactly like sour cream when you dollop it on a baked potato because it is missing that curdled taste, but if you place some inside your bean burrito, it provides enough of a sour cream taste and texture to satisfy most who like sour cream in their food. It is available in most grocery stores. This is a highly processed product, so use sparingly.

Egg Nog

Think you're going to miss your traditional holiday egg nog? Well, I've got good news for you! Silk's Seasonal Nog and So Delicious coconut milk nog taste just like egg nog, just not quite as thick in consistency, which many people prefer. You can find it in most grocery and health food stores during the holiday season. Save this for special occasions.

Whipped Cream

Soyatoo! Whipped Soy Topping is a delicious substitute for whipped cream and can be found in health food stores. Save this for special occasions.

Buttermilk

Stir a tablespoon of white or cider vinegar or lemon juice into a cup of soy milk.

Ice Cream

All of the substitutes are delicious and the variety of flavors continue to expand. They are available in most grocery stores. Save this for special occasions.

Ice Cream Sandwiches

Tofutti Cuties and So Delicious are available in most grocery stores. Save these for special occasions.

Fudgsicles

Tofutti Chocolate Fudge Treats are available in most grocery stores. Save these for special occasions.

For help cooking and baking without eggs and cooking and baking without oil, please refer to those sections within my Helpful Hints chapter. For the ultimate vegan baking cheat sheet, go to this link: http://www.pinterest.com/pin/225954106275817710/.

Soy Protein Isolate

Meat substitutes are great transition foods that make the conversion to a plant-based lifestyle easier. However, they should not become a permanent fixture on your menu. These foods most likely contain soy protein isolate. Soy protein isolate is a highly processed form of soy created by concentrating the protein. Studies have demonstrated that daily consumption of 40 grams of soy protein isolate can carry the same cancer risk and have the same bone draining effect as meat. If you include them in your diet at all past your transition to a low-fat, plant-based lifestyle, treat them as condiments to your meal rather than as a food group, eat them only as an occasional treat, or better yet, eliminate them entirely.

Stocking Your Pantry and Freezer

I always keep a variety of basic non-perishables and quick meals stocked in my pantry and freezer for those days when I don't have time to plan, shop, and cook breakfast, lunch, or dinner. Here are some ideas:

- old fashioned oatmeal cooked with water (or non-dairy milk) and any of the following:
  - fresh, frozen, or dried fruit
  - 100% fruit spread
  - cinnamon
  - pure vanilla extract
  - nuts and/or seeds
  - semi-sweet, non-dairy, chocolate chips
  - topped with 1 tablespoon chia seed, hemp seed, or ground flax seed
- whole grain pancake mixes (make sure they don't contain any dairy) and pure maple syrup
- frozen whole grain waffles
- Amy's frozen Breakfast Burrito
- Amy's frozen Tofu Scramble in a Pocket Sandwich
- low-fat frozen potatoes such as Alexia 98% Fat Free Smart Classics
- low-fat frozen sweet potato fries
- Nabisco Shredded Wheat and Bran, Post Grape-Nuts, Bob's Red Mill Natural Granola (which doesn't contain any added fat), or Post Lightly Sweetened Spoon-Sized Shredded Wheat cereals
- frozen Ezekiel flourless, sprouted whole grain bread, English muffins, buns, and tortillas
- Latin American breakfast (Ezekiel toast topped with rinsed, drained, and heated black beans, salsa, and Dijon mustard)
- natural peanut butter (just peanuts, no added salt or sugar)
- 100% fruit spread
- cocoa

- whole grain muffin mixes
- McDougall's soup cups and soups that are packaged in aseptic cartons
- Progresso 99% Fat Free Lentil Soup
- Amy's Organic Low Fat Split Pea Soup
- Imagine creamy tomato soup
- Tabatchnick frozen vegan soups
- Thai Kitchen Brown Rice Noodles
- Lotus Foods Millet & Brown Rice Ramen is delicious when cooked with a vegan bouillon cube and is a healthier version of Oodles of Noodles
- Thai Kitchen Instant Rice Noodle Soup, Garlic & Vegetable and Spring Onion only, are also healthier versions of Oodles of Noodles
- Amy's canned low-fat bean chili
- Amy's frozen Shepherd's Pie (it should say vegan at the beginning of the ingredients list)
- Amy's frozen Black Bean Vegetable Burrito
- Amy's frozen Bean and Rice Burrito
- Amy's frozen Indian Samosa Wrap
- Amy's has a large number of other 100% plant-based, frozen meals, however, some of their meals do contain cheese. Those products that contain no animal products will indicate that they are vegan at the beginning of the ingredient list.
- ingredients for Black Bean and Salsa Soup
- ingredients for Speedy International Stew
- whole wheat pasta and pasta sauce in a jar such as Prego Light Smart (meatless, cheeseless, and with no/minimal added oil)
- Victoria Vegan's Vegan Vodka Sauce is absolutely delicious and provides those following a plant-based lifestyle with the opportunity to enjoy vodka sauce again (although it has 12 grams of fat per serving so enjoy sparingly or occasionally)!
- brown rice (both long-cooking and pre-cooked Minute Rice brown rice), frozen mixed stir-fry vegetables, and bottled Chinese or Japanese sauce

- frozen Ezekiel whole grain buns, frozen veggie burgers (try to find some without soy protein isolate), Bush's vegetarian baked beans, and a frozen vegetable
- canned Sloppy Joe sauce, frozen Beyond Meat crumbles, frozen French fries or frozen sweet potato fries, and a frozen vegetable
- Mrs. T's Vegan Potato & Onion Pierogies
- frozen vegan Amy's and Tofurky pizzas
- pre-washed quinoa (pronounced keen-wah)
- Near East Whole Grain Blends Brown Rice Pilaf and Wheat Pilaf
- Near East Toasted Pine Nut Couscous
- Kashi 7 Whole Grain Pilaf
- garbanzo, baked, fat-free refried, and other canned beans
- assorted frozen vegetables, fruits, corn, and peas
- raw nuts, seeds, or trail mix such as Aurora Cranberry Health Mix, although limit consumption to ¼ cup per day (store your nuts and seeds in the refrigerator for a longer shelf life)
- flax, chia, and/or hemp seed
  Flax seed needs to be ground before being eaten, otherwise they will pass through you undigested. Either buy the whole seed and use a dedicated coffee grinder immediately before using it or buy it already ground. Store in the freezer (no need to thaw before using) or refrigerator for a longer shelf life.
- wheat germ
- raisins and other dried fruit
- popcorn and lunch-sized brown paper bags to use to pop it in the microwave
- Edward & Sons Brown Rice Snaps (unsalted plain, onion garlic, and tamari sesame flavors) and/or Wasa crisp bread
- Larabars and/or Go Raw Bars (just make sure whatever bars you choose do not contain soy protein isolate)
- 100% frozen fruit bars
- nutritional yeast flakes to sprinkle on pasta, popcorn, etc.
- salsa
- pizza sauce

- banana peppers
- black and green olives
- plant-based gravy
- plant-based bouillon cubes or vegetable broth in aseptic containers
- seasoned rice vinegar to sprinkle on vegetables and grains
- Trader Joe's Fat-Free Balsamic Vinaigrette or other fat-free salad dressings to sprinkle on vegetables and grains
- assortment of your favorite vinegars
- Bragg's Liquid Aminos
- Mrs. Dash
- green tea and/or matcha
- tea bags with hibiscus as the first ingredient
- vitamin B_{12}

For a visual view of some of my favorite plant-based products, go to my Pinterest board, So What Should I Eat?: http://pinterest.com/traceyeakin/so-what-should-i-eat/.

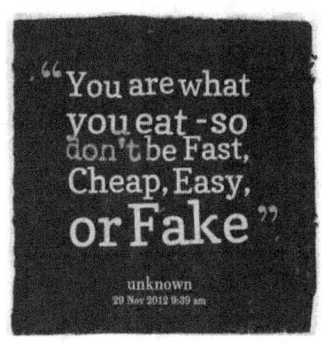

Tips for a Healthy Shopping Trip

Refer to my chapter Stocking Your Pantry and Freezer and this chapter, Tips for a Healthy Shopping Trip, as you create your shopping list.

Always strive to eat plant food as close to its naturally packaging as possible. The less processed/refined the food is, the better. As a general rule, packaged and processed food may not be in a form recognizable by your body, it likely contains added sugar, fat, and salt, and probably includes artificial preservatives and other chemicals designed to increase its shelf life. It may also have refined grains that have been stripped of their nutritious germ and bran layers.

That said, there are some packaged foods that can be used that won't sacrifice your health, should help save time, and should make this lifestyle easier to adopt:

Frozen Vegetables – Vegetables are the most nutrient dense food and an important component of a healthy lifestyle. Frozen vegetables are not only extremely convenient, they may also be more nutritious than their fresh counterparts. Vegetables begin to lose their nutrients as soon as they are picked. Frozen vegetables are supposedly picked at their peak ripeness, then quickly frozen, thereby locking in their nutrition. Depending upon where your fresh vegetables are grown, the time it takes to get them from the farm to your grocery store, the amount of time they sit in the store and then in your home after you purchase them, to when they are finally eaten, can vary greatly.

Just be careful to select frozen vegetables that do not contain any added ingredients such as sauces. Some contain added salt, but they usually meet the guideline for added salt, which is explained in the next chapter on reading labels. Keep many different varieties on hand for quick and easy access to nature's gold mine of nutrition. I prefer not to microwave my vegetables in those "steam-in-bags".

Frozen Fruit – Keep a variety of frozen fruit for the same reasons. In addition, frozen fruit can be used to make smoothies, plant-based ice creams, and other desserts ice cold. Why add just ice cubes to make something cold when you can accomplish the same effect with frozen fruit and add additional nutrition at the same time? Don't forget to freeze your own fresh fruit and vegetables if you don't think you will be able to eat them before they spoil. Both can be thrown into smoothies, especially frozen bananas, and vegetables can be added to soups, stews, and sauces.

Intact Whole Grains – Minimally processed whole grains, legumes, and starchy vegetables should comprise 80% of the food that we consume. They breakdown into glucose, our body's preferred primary source of fuel. Always keep a variety of intact whole grains on hand such as old fashioned oatmeal, farro, brown rice, barley, corn, quinoa (even though quinoa is technically a seed), and millet.

Quick Cooking Brown Rice – I always keep a box or two of Minute Rice Brown Rice in my pantry, alongside my assortment of long-cooking rices because despite my best efforts, there will undoubtedly be days when I'm too short on time to make rice from scratch. The rice itself is still unadulterated. It has just been pre-cooked and dehydrated. When you make it, you're just rehydrating it.

Whole Grain Pasta – Keep your favorite varieties of whole grain pasta and jars of your favorite sauce on hand for a healthy meal that can be prepared quickly and at the last minute.

Most processed grains, even processed whole grains, like bread, bagels, tortillas, dry cereal, pretzels, crackers, and other flour products, are very calorie dense. Whole grain pasta is processed, but is not as calorie dense because of the water that the pasta absorbs as it is being cooked. This water lowers its overall calorie density and increases the satiety that it provides.

Canned Beans – Next to vegetables, beans are one of the most nutrient dense foods we can eat. They are also packed with fiber which makes them a very filling food. However, dried beans can take hours to soak and cook and are not a reasonable option for last minute meals. Luckily, a wide variety of canned beans are readily available at the grocery store. Look for beans without any added salt and without BPA, a carcinogen, sprayed on the inside of the can. Eden beans are BPA-free and are available at most grocery stores.

Canned Tomatoes - Canned tomatoes can provide the base for many quick meals. Try to find tomatoes without added salt and in a can that has not been sprayed with BPA. Pomi brand are both salt and BPA-free. Some tomato products are available in aseptic containers as well.

Perishables - As the name implies, these foods will need to be purchased more often since they do indeed have a shorter shelf life:

Select a variety of fresh vegetables and fruits. Try not to buy more than you think you'll eat and don't be afraid to try something new. The internet is a great resource when you are exploring how to cook a new vegetable or fruit. Always try to include dark green, leafy vegetables as they are nutrition super stars and a great source for calcium and iron.

Other perishables include non-dairy milk, yogurt, and coffee creamer; low-fat hummus; low-fat guacamole; and whole wheat Boboli shells for homemade pizza.

In general, don't grocery shop when you are hungry.

Plan your purchases ahead of time with a list to better avoid unhealthy, impulse purchases.

Partially hydrogenated vegetable oils, also known as trans fats, are as bad as saturated fats. Avoid them.

Michael Greger, MD recommends greens, beans, berries, green tea, and nuts every day.

Mastering Label Reading

Although I don't recommend processed food, sometimes it is difficult to avoid it completely. It is much easier to interpret ingredient lists when they only have one or two ingredients. When you buy a bag of brown rice, the ingredient list will likely only contain one ingredient - brown rice. This makes choosing healthy food pretty easy. When that is not possible, you need to be to be able to chose products that are health promoting and avoid products that are damaging to your health.

Two words simplify the process of determining if the food contains any animal products. If you find pareve or vegan on a food label, your job is done. The product contains no animal products.

Listed below are ingredients to avoid:

Dairy Derivatives - beta-lactoglobulin, casein, caseinate (ammonium caseinate, calcium caseinate, magnesium caseinate, potassium caseinate, and sodium caseinate), ghee, kefir, lactalbumin and lactalbumin phosphate lactoferrin, lactose, whey

Egg Derivatives - Albumin/albumen, conalbumin, Egg Beaters®, globulin, livetin, lysozyme, meringue, ovalbumin, ovoglobulin, ovolactohydrolyze proteins, ovomacroglobulin, ovomucin, ovomucoid, ovotransferrin, ovovitellin, silico-albuminate, Simplesse®, vitellin

Other Items of Animal Origin - diglycerides, gelatin, honey, lactic acid, lard, lecithin, monoglycerides, rennet, tallow

Fat - diglycerides, lard, monoglycerides, tallow

Sugar - barley malt, cane juice crystals, corn syrup, corn syrup solids, dextran, dextrose, diastatic malt, diastase, ethyl maltol, fructose, galactose, glucose, high fructose corn syrup, lactose, maltodextrin, maltose, malt syrup, maple syrup, molasses, panocha, refiner's syrup, rice syrup, sorbitol, sorghum syrup, sucrose, sugar, treacle, turbinado sugar

If something is characterized as a natural source, it can be of animal, vegetable, or mineral origin.

Although the following ingredients may sound like they are of an animal origin, they are not: calcium and sodium lactate, calcium and sodium stearoyl lactylate, cocoa butter, cream of tartar, oleoresin

I'm also going to share with you some tips from a trusted source of mine, Jeff Novick, MS, RD, LD, LN. Listed below are Jeff's guidelines for evaluating if a product is healthy for you and discerning between a product's nutrition information and its advertisements.

Rule #1: Never, ever believe anything on the front of the product...ever! It's purely advertising and marketing.

Rule #2: Always read the nutrition facts label and the ingredient list.

Nutrition Facts

Serving Size: 8 OZ./ 227 grams

Amount Per Serving

Calories 60	Calories From Fat 15

	% Daily Value*
Total Fat 1.5g	**3%**
Saturated Fat 0g	**1%**
Trans Fat 0g	
Cholesterol 0mg	**0%**
Sodium 710mg	**30%**
Total Carbohydrate 11g	**4%**
Dietary Fiber 2g	**9%**
Sugars 4g	
Protein 2g	

Vitamin A 50%	• Vitamin C 20%
Calcium 4%	• Iron 4%

* Percent Daily Values are based on a 2,000 calorie diet. Your daily values may be higher or lower depending on your calorie needs:

		Calories	2,000	2,500
Total Fat	Less than		65g	80g
Sat Fat	Less than		20g	25g
Cholesterol	Less than		300mg	300mg
Sodium	Less than		2,400mg	2,400mg
Total Carbohydrate			300g	375g
Dietary Fiber			25g	30g

Rule #3: Calories from fat should not be more than 25% of the total calories per serving in packaged foods. Eliminate saturated animal fats (lard, butter, chicken fat, dairy, cheese), minimize saturated vegetable fat (coconut oil, cocoa butter, palm oil, palm kernel oil), and avoid manmade saturated vegetable fat (partially hydrogenated vegetable oil also known as trans fat, margarine, and shortening). Your body only needs 3%-5% of your calories to come from fat and that can easily be obtained from the plant kingdom.

In the nutrition facts label depicted above, divide the calories from fat by the total calories per serving and multiply by 100: (15 / 60) * 100 = 25%.

Rule #4: If you are eating a minimally processed, low-fat, plant-based lifestyle, your daily fiber goal should be 72 grams (25 grams of soluble fiber and 47 grams of insoluble fiber), with a minimum amount of 40-50 grams. If you are incorporating enough beans into your day, 72 grams is reasonably attainable.

Rule #5: The sodium per serving should be equal to or less than the calories per serving. For example, if the calories per serving are 220, then to be acceptable, the sodium should not exceed 220 mg. Your daily sodium intake should be less than 2,000 mg per day.

You may have guessed that the nutrition facts label pictured above is for a canned vegetable soup as the sodium content is much higher than the 60 mg limit for a food with 60 calories per serving.

Rule #6: For foods that will fill you up without a huge investment in calories, choose foods that contain fewer calories per serving than grams of weight per serving. You want the weight of the food to fill you up before the calories in that food fill you out! Airy foods such as melba toast, pretzels, and bread are not especially high in calories, but will not fill you up either.

In the example above, one serving of the vegetable soup weighs 227 grams and contains 60 calories. The weight in grams, 227, is greater than the calories per serving, 60, so this food should fill you up before its calories fill you out. You will notice this is the case for most soups, making them good choices from this perspective.

Rule #7: Try to avoid foods that have sugar (see list above) in the first three to five ingredients.

Rule #8: Choose whole grains over refined grains. Look for the word "whole", spelled just like that, or rolled in the case of oats. These represent whole grains. Organic, unbleached semolina and wheat flour are other names for refined, white flour. If there are at least 3 g of fiber per 100 calories, that is a good indication that it's made with whole grains.

Eating Out

Eating out doesn't have to be an intimidating event to be avoided. It can be just as enjoyable as it has always been and it doesn't have to sabotage all of your effort and progress.

Social Events

Navigating social events is easy with a little planning and some simple strategies:

- Offer to bring a dish. That way, you can be assured of having something low-fat and plant-based to eat. If you bring a casserole that contains most of the food groups, you'll be covered even if there is nothing else at the party to eat.
- Avoid starving yourself the day of the event in an effort to store up extra calories. You risk arriving at the party too hungry to be able to make prudent decisions about what to eat. Eat moderately throughout the day.
- A host/hostess is less likely to repeatedly try to feed you if you carry a token plate containing some vegetables, fruit, or whatever you brought to the party.

Restaurants

Try to eat home-cooked meals as much as possible, at least at the very beginning. It provides you with the most control over what you eat and how it is prepared. However, whether out of necessity or desire, you do go to a restaurant, it is usually possible to find meals that are in line with your new lifestyle. Here are some strategies for eating out:

- If you are picking the restaurant or weighing in on where to go, consider patronizing a plant-based restaurant or a restaurant that offers plant-based meals that are clearly identified on their menus. If you are located in Pittsburgh, go to www.VeganPittsburgh.org for a comprehensive list of possible locations. If you are not in Pittsburgh or are on vacation, I highly recommend www.HappyCow.net or http://www.VeganEatingOut.com/restaurants/. If you find a restaurant that is not on VeganPittsburgh.org, please email them so that it can be added. If you find a restaurant not listed on HappyCow.net, they encourage you to add it so that their listings are as comprehensive as possible.

Just keep in mind that vegan does not always equate to healthy. Added oils and meat analogs may be vegan, but they do not promote optimal health.

- If you are going to a restaurant that doesn't serve just plant-based food, then take a look at their menu posted on their web site ahead of time.

    1. Look for entrees that are free of animal products and minimal in added oil.
    2. If there aren't any, look for entrees that look good that you can ask if the meat could be left out and possibly replaced with something else and that can be prepared with minimal added oil.
    3. If there don't appear to be any entrees that would work, take a look at the appetizers, side dishes, or the sides that accompany the meat-based entrees. Appetizers can often be prepared as entrées and there will often be some sort of potato, rice, pasta, bean, or winter squash sides and a variety of vegetables. Select an assortment of side dishes that look tasty.
    4. If you still don't see anything that appeals to you, contact the restaurant a few days ahead of time, during non-peak hours, and ask if there is a plant-based meal with no/minimal oil that could be made for you. Most chefs welcome the chance to be

creative and make something out of the ordinary, and they appreciate the extra time so that they can procure the right ingredients. Even if you don't have the ability to call ahead, the restaurant will almost assuredly be able to make something for you. Don't be afraid to ask your server. Some of my best meals have been complete surprises.

Ethnic restaurants are often good choices for eating out.

Italian restaurants have pasta dishes with vegetables and marinara sauce. Make sure that their pasta isn't made with eggs. If it is, most restaurants will keep eggless pasta in the kitchen to accommodate those that cannot eat eggs. Order bread and ask for roasted garlic or a side of marinara sauce for dipping instead of butter or olive oil.

Mexican restaurants will often have bean burritos. Ask if it can be made with whole beans. If that isn't possible, make sure that their refried beans do not contain lard. They may, however, contain added oil. Opt for corn tortillas instead of flour tortillas, which are made with oil. Better yet, you can create a delicious meal by asking for brown rice, beans, grilled vegetables, and guacamole on a bed of romaine lettuce. Ask for warm corn tortillas to dip in salsa in place of fried chips. Mad Mex can make any of their menu items with tofu or portabella mushrooms instead of meat and offers vegan substitutes for cheese, sour cream, and ranch salad dressing, although consider adding them to your meal sparingly or only occasionally as these vegan alternatives are not low in fat.

Chinese restaurants have steamed mixed vegetables over brown rice and plenty of noodle dishes. Just remember to ask them to omit the fried egg and go light on or omit the oil.

Japanese restaurants have miso soup, vegetarian sushi (Futo Maki, Horenso, Kappa Maki, Oshinko Roll, and Kamp), udon vegetable soup (ask for it to be made without any animal products), cucumber salad, sunomono salad, and edamame (soybeans). If you want to order a seaweed salad, make sure their salad does not contain jellyfish.

Thai restaurants often offer green papaya salad, noodles, and steamed rice. Just be mindful of the dishes that contain coconut and/or coconut milk as they tend to be higher in fat.

Indian restaurants always have dishes that include potatoes, lentils, split peas, garbanzo beans, and cauliflower. Just be careful that the dish you order does not contain cheese, a dairy-based sauce, or a lot of oil. Choose aloo gobi (potatoes and cauliflower), chana pindi (garbanzo beans), or pulao rice. Hold the naan as it is fried bread made from white flour. Opt instead for two other Indian breads: tandoori roti and onion kulcha. Ask them to hold the ghee and opt for mango chutney instead.

If you go to a traditional American restaurant, you might find success in ordering a selection of side dishes if there aren't any entrees that meet your needs. Some restaurants now have veggie burgers that can be coupled with a baked potato and side salad. To avoid the refined carbohydrates such as bread, buns, and wraps usually offered in restaurants, try asking for the sandwich or wrap contents on a bed of greens instead. Ask for sauces and salad dressings on the side and then use sparingly. Some pizza parlors now offer whole wheat crusts that can be topped with extra tomato sauce and plenty of vegetables. In many restaurants, you can order fresh fruit or sorbet for dessert. Don't forget to ask for water with lemon or lime wedges instead of pop.

Here are some Pittsburgh restaurants that provide low-fat, plant-based options:

Loving Hut, 5474 Campbells Run Road, Pittsburgh, PA 15205, 412-787-2727, www.lovinghut.us/pittsburgh_01 is a delicious, entirely plant-based, restaurant. They have an all-you-can-eat buffet once a month. I highly recommend it. They are not open on Sunday.

The Zenith Vegetarian Cafe, 86 South 26th Street, Pittsburgh, PA 15203, 412-481-4833, www.zenithpgh.com

Tin Front Cafe, 216 East Eighth Avenue, Homestead, PA 15120, 412-461-4615, http://tinfrontcafe.weebly.com/, their menu is on their Facebook page, https://www.facebook.com/tinfrontcafe

Eden, 735 Copeland Street, Pittsburgh, PA (Shadyside), 412-802-7070, hello@edenpitt.com, http://www.edenpitt.com/

Double Wide Grill, 2339 East Carson Street, Pittsburgh, PA 15203, 412-390-1111, www.doublewidegrill.com

Eleven, Mad Mex's sister restaurant, always has a vegetarian tasting menu, which can be prepared vegan upon request, http://www.elevenck.com/

Kaya, another Big Burrito restaurant, holds a monthly vegetarian prix fixe. Depending upon the menu planned for that month, they may be able to make it vegan. Just call the restaurant to make sure first. Reservations are recommended, 412-261-6565. http://www.bigburrito.com/kaya/index.shtml

Randita's Vegan Cafe, 210 West Main Street, Saxonburg, PA 16056, 724-822-8677, http://www.randitas.com/

Casa Rasta, 2056 Broadway Avenue, Pittsburgh, PA 15216, 412-344-4700, http://www.casarastapgh.com/, tacos and Caribbean fusion

Spak Brothers Pizza and More, 5107 Penn Avenue, Pittsburgh, PA 15224, 412-362-7725, http://www.spakbrothers.com, seitan wings; vegan cheese, seitan, portabella mushroom, and tempeh hoagies; vegan pizzas; seitan salads; vegetarian tacos

Piper's Pub and Pub Chip Shop (next door), 1828 East Carson Street, Pittsburgh, PA 15203, 412-381-3977, http://piperspub.com/, they do a vegan soup, vegetarian lunch, and vegan dinner at both places every Tuesday and keep vegan items on their menus year round

Fortuitea Cafe, The Shoppes at Quail Acres, 1445 Washington Road, Washington, PA 15301, http://www.fortuiteacafe.com/, all vegan cafe and bakery

Jacksons Restaurant - Rotisserie - Bar, Southpointe and Moon Township, https://www.experiencejacksons.com/, because of customer demand, they always have a plant-based option on their menu

Taza 21, 1827 Murray Avenue, Pittsburgh, PA 15217, 412-904-2764

Lili Coffee Shop, 3138 Dobson Street, Pittsburgh, PA 15219, 412-682-3600

Fast Food Restaurants

In today's hectic world, fast food is a necessary evil for some, but it doesn't have to set you back on your course to a more healthful life. Keep in mind that this is not optimal eating and the less frequently you need to rely on fast food for your meals, the better.

For a comprehensive, online guide to plant-based fast food options, refer to the following link: http://www.veganeatingout.com/fast-food/. Here are some options that I have found:

Chipotle Mexican Grill, http://chipotle.com/home

> Burrito Bowl-your choice of brown and/or cilantro-lime rice, vegetarian black and/or pinto beans, fajita vegetables, romaine lettuce, guacamole, and salsa (fresh tomato salsa, roasted chili-corn salsa, tomatillo-green chili salsa, and tomatillo-red chili salsa)

> Burrito-everything available in a burrito bowl but wrapped in a flour tortilla

Moe's Southwest Grill, http://www.moes.com/

Subway, http://www.subway.com/subwayroot/default.aspx

> Veggie Delight Sub-your choice of lettuce, tomatoes, green peppers, black olives, and onion with your choice of fat-free condiments on freshly baked bread, available in 6" or 12"

> Veggie Delight Salad-the same as the Veggie Delight Sub without the sub

> Apple Slices

Taco Bell, http://www.tacobell.com/

> Bean Burrito, 1/2 lb. Cheesy Bean & Rice Burrito (hold the cheese), 7-Layer Burrito (hold the cheese and sour cream), ordered Fresco Style (replaces the sauce and cheese with fiesta salsa, a freshly prepared blend of tomatoes, diced white onions, and cilantro)

> Sides-Black Beans & Rice, Mexican Rice, Pintos N Cheese (hold the cheese), and Cheesy Fiesta Potatoes (hold the cheese and sour cream)

> Their beans do not contain lard.

Burger King, http://www.bk.com/

> Breakfast-oatmeal and apple slices

> Lunch/Dinner-BK Veggie burger (does contain milk and eggs, but in an absolute pinch, is better than its high-fat, animal-based alternative), garden side salad (hold the cheese), and apple slices

Wendy's, https://www.wendys.com/

baked potato(es) but hold the cheese, sour cream, and bacon and instead top with fat-free or low-fat salad dressing, with garden side salad and apple slices

Papa Johns, http://www.papajohns.com/index.html

Your choice of green peppers, baby portabella mushrooms, roma tomatoes, jalapeño peppers, onions, black olives, pineapple, and banana peppers (hold the cheese)

Sheetz, https://www.sheetz.com/

Made-to-Order Food

Veggie Wrap - your choice of rice and beans, lettuce, tomatoes, onions, green peppers, pickles, black olives, mild pepper rings, jalapeños, salt, pepper, oregano, ketchup, yellow mustard, fire roasted tomato sauce, BBQ sauce, buffalo sauce, and habanera sauce

Garden Salad - romaine lettuce, rice and beans, tomatoes, green peppers, onions, black olives, pickles, mild pepper rings, jalapeño peppers, croutons, salt, pepper, buffalo sauce, and crackers

Veggie Sandwich - wheat bread, your choice of veggies listed above, ketchup, mustard, BBQ sauce, buffalo sauce, habanera sauce

Sides - rice and beans, apple slices

Other Choices - Dole fruit in 100% fruit juice, garden salads, fresh cut fruit and vegetables, and bottled water

VeganABC, http://www.veganabc.com/, a stall in the Strip District's Pittsburgh Public Market

Bakeries

Bella Christie and Lil Z's Sweet Boutique, bakery with vegan selections, 213 Commercial Avenue, Aspinwall, PA 15215, 412-772-1283, http://www.asweetboutique.com/

Gluuteny Bakery • gluten free • casein free • and sometimes vegan, 1923 Murray Avenue, Pittsburgh, PA 15217, 412-521-4890, info@gluuteny.com, http://www.gluuteny.com/

Eden restaurant in Shadyside also offers their desserts to go, http://www.edenpitt.com.

Fortuitea Cafe, The Shoppes at Quail Acres, 1445 Washington Road, Washington, PA 15301, http://www.fortuiteacafe.com/, all vegan cafe and bakery

Sunny Bridge Natural Foods in Peters Township usually carries vegan, palm oil-free cupcakes, http://www.sunnybridgenaturalfoods.com/.

Allison's Gourmet, a vegan bakery and confectionery boutique: www.allisonsgourmet.com

Potlucks

To find plant-based potlucks, as well as other events and local, kindred support, go to http://www.meetup.com and search plant-based, vegan, or other related term, to locate groups and events in your area. There is one in Pittsburgh: The Pittsburgh Vegan Meetup.

Brown Bag Lunches

Many of the meal ideas in this book are portable. Many of the recipes included in this book can be made to go.

If you have access to a microwave, the following items can be purchased at a grocery store and heated up for a quick, healthy meal:

Minute Ready to Serve! in Brown & Wild Rice, Jasmine Rice, Multi-Grain Medley, and Brown Rice

Uncle Ben's Ready Whole Grain Medley Pouch in Vegetable Harvest, Santa Fe, and Brown Basmati

Roland Israeli Cous Cous and Quinoa (leave out the oil)

If you don't have access to a microwave, or if you travel a lot and find yourself eating out of your car, here are a few more ideas:

fresh fruit

individual containers of 100% applesauce

sliced vegetables

pull top cans of garbanzo beans

Read Southwestern Bean Salad (can opener required)

zip lock bag of spoon-sized shredded wheat, Bob's Red Mill Natural Granola (which doesn't contain any added fat), or Post lightly sweetened spoon-sized shredded wheat

bag of small red potatoes microwaved and refrigerated the night before (just eat them like apples)

raw nuts and seeds

trail mix of raw nuts, seeds, and dried fruit (such as Aurora Natural Cranberry Health Mix)

brown rice cakes

previously refrigerated container of cooked frozen corn mixed with your favorite beans and salsa or fat-free balsamic vinaigrette

If you travel a lot, you may want to consider purchasing a travel cooler/warmer. It plugs into the power outlet of your car. An electrical outlet adapter can be purchased for use when you reach your final destination.

You may also want to scope out any Whole Foods Markets, Trader Joe's, Giant Eagle Market Districts, or health food stores along your travel route or at your destination so that you can plan to eat there and/or stock up on foods that you can eat along the way and/or keep in your hotel room. Check www.localharvest.org to find farmers markets and www.greenpages.org to find co-ops, health food stores, and green businesses.

Plant-Based Meal Delivery Services

Pittsburgh-based Chip and Kale, http://chipandkale.com/

Veestro, http://www.veestro.com/

Nirvana Kitchen, http://nirvanakitchen.com/

Greenlite Meals, www.greenlitemeals.com or 1-800-684-7618.

Plant-Based Catering Services

Bistro To Go & Company, http://bistroandcompany.com/

Here is the link to their plant-based offerings: http://bistroandcompany.com/wp-content/uploads/2014/02/BTG-Vegetarian-Catering-Menu-2014.pdf

All in Good Taste Productions, www.allingoodtasteproductions.com

Miscellaneous Adventures

For those who are really adventurous, look into the following vegan cruise!

www.atasteofhealth.org/vegan-cruise.htm

If you live in Pittsburgh, you are very fortunate to live so close to the annual conference of the North American Vegetarian Society. Each summer, they hold their Vegetarian Summerfest in Johnstown, PA. The link to the event is: http://vegetariansummerfest.org/.

There are Veg Fests held all over the country. Search the internet for one near you.

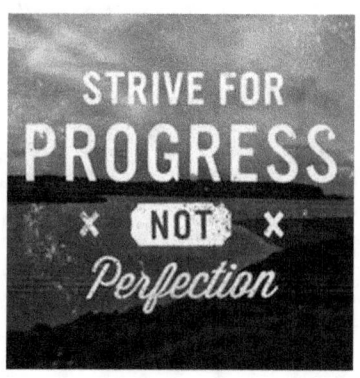

Helpful Hints

This section contains a variety of suggestions that I've accumulated over the years to help my clients.

General Recommendations

- Contrary to what was once thought, it is not necessary to combine certain foods within one meal, such as rice and beans, in order to ensure that we consume all of the essential amino acids. As long as we eat a variety of whole, plant foods on a regular basis, our bodies will be able to acquire all of the essential amino acids. However, certain combinations have been found to be greater than the sum of their parts:
    - Eating fat with plants can maximize the absorption of certain important phytonutrients. It's best to try to use fat from whole plant foods like nuts, nut butters, seeds, olives, avocados, coconut, and full-fat tofu. For example, salad dressings made with tahini (ground sesame seeds) or nuts and seeds added to a salad, can increase the absorption of the phytonutrients of the plants in the salad. Only 5 walnut halves or ¼ of an avocado are all that we need to maximize absorption.

Try adding guacamole to salsa for a phytonutrient boost.

- o The whole grain phytonutrient, phytic acid (phytate), partially inhibits mineral absorption, but has a wide-range of health-promoting properties such as anti-cancer activity. By concurrently eating mineral absorption enhancers such as garlic and onions (in fact, anything from the allium family), one can get the best of both worlds by improving the bioavailability of iron and zinc in plant foods.
- o The active ingredient in turmeric, curcumin, has very poor bioavailability unless consumed with black pepper, which increases its absorption by 2000%.

- Vegetable stocks can be created by blending any cooked vegetables including broccoli and asparagus stems.
- Frozen hash browns add body and instant mashed potatoes thicken soups and stews.
- If you find certain green vegetables to be too bitter to be palatable, such as broccoli or spinach, try sprinkling a bit of lemon juice on them.
- A balsamic reduction, balsamic vinegar boiled down, can be drizzled over vegetables, potatoes, etc. Any vinegar cooked down will turn out sweet.
- Place leftover bean and vegetable dishes in corn or wheat tortillas and freeze for future use. Top with enchilada, marinara, curry, or salsa sauce and reheat in the microwave for a quick but healthy meal.
- Mirin is a Japanese condiment. It is a kind of rice wine and is used as a substitute for sugar and soy sauce. Only a small amount is used as it has a very strong flavor. Tofu slices and be mixed with mirin and grilled or stir-fried.
- Agar-agar and Emes Kosher Gelatin can be used in place of gelatin in molded salad recipes.

- If you are new to beans, start with small amounts and be sure they are well cooked to avoid indigestion. If you cook with dried beans, make sure to replace the soaking water with fresh water prior to cooking.
- If beans appear to give you excessive gas, there are some steps you can take to relieve your distress:
    - Lentils, split peas, and canned beans tend to produce less gas. Tofu does not appear to be an offender at all.
    - If you soak your own dried beans, try adding 1/16 of a teaspoon of baking soda to your soaking water. Make sure to drain off the soaking water, rinse your beans well several times, and then use fresh water to cook them.
    - The more you eat beans, the more your body will adapt to them, at least to a certain extent.
    - For those of you that continue to be bothered, don't avoid beans, just take Beano before eating them. It contains the enzyme alpha-galactosidase, which will break down the previously indigestible bean sugars.
    - The same holds true for cruciferous vegetables like broccoli, cabbage, and Brussels sprouts. Take it easy at first until your body adapts to the new food.
- Per Michael Greger, MD the biggest nutrition bang for your buck is broccoli sprouts. Soak 1 tablespoon of broccoli seeds in filtered water overnight in a seed jar (or a Mason jar with a screen over the mouth), drain them in the morning, then rinse them twice daily. This will generate about 2 cups of broccoli sprouts in 4-5 days. Rotate sprouting jars so that you have a constant supply. Dr. Greger does not recommend alfalfa sprouts (even when home sprouted) as fecal bacteria from manure can hide in the seed's nooks and crannies and cause illness. The second biggest nutrition bang for your buck is red/purple cabbage. Keep some in your refrigerator's crisper and slice off shreds for use in whatever you are cooking/eating.

- Dr. Greger also recommends keeping a container of rinsed & drained beans in the fridge to spoon into whatever you happen to be eating throughout the day.
- Michael Greger, MD, recommends eating mushrooms after they've been cooked as there is a natural toxin found in them called agaratine, which is destroyed by cooking.
- How many nuts comprise one ounce of tree nuts? The answer depends upon the nut:

Almonds: 20-24 nuts

Brazil nuts: 6-8 nuts

Cashews: 16-18 nuts

Hazelnuts: 18-20 nuts

Macadamias: 10-12 nuts

Pecans: 18-20 halves

Pine nuts: 150-157nuts

Pistachios: 47-49 nuts

Walnuts: 8-14 halves

- To chop fresh parsley quickly, place the sprigs in a large measuring cup and snip with clean kitchen shears.
- Drop pasta into boiling water a little at a time so that the water does not stop boiling. If you are planning on serving it hot with sauce, drain it but do not rinse it in cold water which removes the starch on the pasta that encourages the sauce to stick to it. If however you are using the pasta cold in a salad, when it is done cooking, drain it and rinse it in cold water.

- Avocados discolor when exposed to air. To keep mashed avocado looking fresher longer, place the pit in the bowl with the avocado and cover with plastic wrap.

- Toasting heightens the aroma, flavor, and crispness of nuts, seeds, and rice. To toast nuts and seeds, place them in a single layer on an unoiled baking sheet in an oven or toaster oven at 350 degrees F until they're fragrant and lightly browned (about 5 minutes for most nuts and a couple of minutes for seeds). I place a piece of parchment paper between my nuts and seeds and my toaster oven tray as it is aluminum. For rice, you can usually toast it in the dry pot that you plan to cook it in once you add the water. Try adding barley to the rice and cook them together.

- To soften aging breads, bagels, and tortillas, place them in the microwave on high for 15-45 seconds.

- To keep from crying when chopping onions, breathe only through your nose. Do not talk or open your mouth at all.

- To find a plant-based substitute for any baking need, check out this fabulous infographic:

http://www.pinterest.com/pin/225954106275817710/

Cooking/Baking Without Eggs

Replacing eggs in recipes is easy, and if you can determine the purpose of the eggs in the recipe, then you can select what would serve as the best substitute. There are three main reasons for adding eggs to recipes. They might be included for binding, for leavening (to make the final product light and fluffy), or to add moistness. The following list, provided by vegan chef Isa Chandra Moskowitz, will provide you with several alternatives. Each is the equivalent of one egg:

For Binding:

2 tablespoons of flaxseed meal plus 3 tablespoons of water

2 tablespoons of cornstarch plus 2 tablespoons of water

¼ cup pureed silken tofu

¼ cup soy yogurt

¼ cup applesauce

½ ripe banana, mashed

¼ cup pureed fruit

For Leavening:

1 teaspoon baking powder plus 1 tablespoon white vinegar

2 teaspoons baking soda plus 2 tablespoons water

2 tablespoons potato starch plus 2 tablespoons water

For Moisture:

¼ cup pureed silken tofu

¼ cup applesauce

¼ cup pureed fruit

To replace eggs in meatless loaves and veggie burgers, tomato paste, mashed potato, moistened bread crumbs, or rolled oats can be used in their place.

Here is the link to my video, "Baking Without Eggs": www.youtube.com/watch?v=eyg8PqJUnIs.

Cooking/Baking Without Oil

The cookware you choose to use is very important. Heating the cookware can cause your food to pick up molecules from your cookware, utensils, and the material you use to cover your food such as aluminum foil. Aluminum cookware should be avoided. Instead, opt for glass, glass coated with silicon, stainless steel, any of the new, non-Teflon, non-stick cookware, silicon-coated bake ware, solid silicon bake ware, and porcelain. Parchment paper can be placed between metal bake ware, including baking sheets, and your food and can be placed between your food and aluminum foil. Silicone baking mats can be used to help keep food from sticking on baking sheets and in the bottom of traditional bake ware.

Whenever a recipe calls for oiling a baking dish, I've never done it and have never found it to be a problem. It's suggested so that it's easier to remove the food when it's done cooking and so that it's easier to clean the dish afterward, but I've never found a plant-based meal that is anywhere close to the headache of cleaning up a meat and dairy (especially cheese)-based meal. I also use paper baking cups in my muffin tins to make getting the muffins out and cleaning up the tins even easier. If vegetables stick while cooking in a pan or baking tray or if you baked muffins without the muffin cups and they are sticking, try letting both cool first for about 5 to 10 minutes.

To cook pancakes without fat, use a non-stick griddle or pan and just before ladling the batter onto the cooking surface, sprinkle a small amount of the dry mix onto the cooking surface.

Guar gum can be used to thicken homemade salad dressing in place of oil. Stir it into the dressing and it will thicken in one hour without heating.

Vegetables do not need to be sautéed in oil to be tasty. Try sautéing in a small amount of:

- water
- vegetable broth
- red or white wine (alcoholic or non-alcoholic)
- sherry (alcoholic or non-alcoholic)
- Bragg Liquid Aminos, tamari, or soy sauce
- vegan Worcestershire sauce
- oil-free salad dressing
- barbeque sauce mixed with a little water
- rice or balsamic vinegar
- fruit juice
- salsa
- tomato juice
- lemon or lime juice
- water with herbs and spices, such as gingerroot, dry mustard, or garlic

When cooking without added fat, use fresh herbs instead of dried herbs. Dried herbs need the oil to release their flavor and aroma. If dried herbs are all that are available, more may need to be used than stated in the recipe. Try growing your own herbs. It is easy and much less expensive than buying them.

Crushing herbs releases flavor. Crush dried herbs by holding them in the palm of one hand and crushing them with the fingers of your other hand or try using a mortar and pestle for hard herbs and seeds.

1 tablespoon of fresh = 1 teaspoon of dried for most herbs.

Use kosher or sea salt instead of regular salt. They dissolve better. They can also be sprinkled on slightly damp vegetables in place of oil so that spices adhere to vegetables that are going to be roasted.

A roux is a flour and butter (or other fat) mixture used as a gravy or to thicken sauces and soups. A corn starch slurry can be used instead by mixing equal parts of cornstarch and water. Arrowroot, tapioca flour, potato flour, and soy flour can also act as thickening agents. Start by boiling a vegetable-based liquid, perhaps onion and water, then add the slurry and spices.

To replace oil or butter in baked goods and desserts, substitute **with half the amount** called for in the recipe with one of the following foods:

- applesauce
- mashed bananas
- fig or prune puree (recipe provided below)
- mashed potatoes
- mashed pumpkin
- tomato sauce
- soft silken tofu
- soy yogurt

Baked goods prepared without oil are usually heavier than their traditional counterpart. For a lighter texture, replace water with carbonated water in baking recipes. Keep in mind that oil-free baked goods may need to bake a little longer than stated in the recipe, depending upon the weather and altitude in which you live.

Prune Puree

From Mary McDougall

Preparation Time: 10 minutes

Servings: makes about 3 ½ cups

2 cups dried pitted plums (prunes)

warm water

In a glass 4-cup measuring container, add 2 cups of dried plums (prunes), up to the 2-cup mark. Make sure none of them have pits in them. Do not remove them. Add warm water up to the 4-cup mark. Let it rest for 3-5 minutes. Then, place the contents of the container into a high speed blender or food processor (if you do not have a large food processor, this can be done in batches). Process until the mixture is the consistency of applesauce. Cover and refrigerate until ready to use.

This will keep in the refrigerator for about 2 weeks, but can also be frozen in smaller amounts for use in future recipes, perhaps in ½ cup increments. It will keep for at least a year in the freezer, just remember to provide enough time for it to thaw before it is needed in your recipe. This can be used in brownies, pancakes, muffins, etc., whenever a good substitute for fat is needed in baked goods.

Think outside the box when minimizing added oils. Instead of adding butter, margarine, or Earth Balance organic buttery spread (my recommendation for a butter substitute), try topping baked potatoes or eggless noodles with fat-free Italian salad dressing or even vegetarian baked beans. It keeps the starch from tasting dry and prevents you from having to add additional fat.

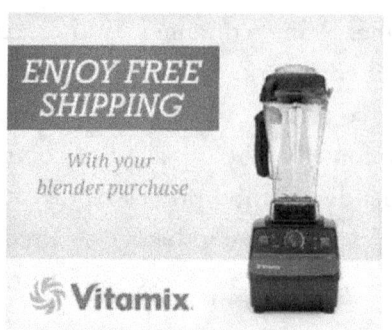
Vitamix
An Investment in Your Health and the Health of Your Loved Ones

Vitamix is the gold standard in high performance blending machines. I purchased the Vitamix 5200 Super-Healthy Lifestyle model as well as the Live Fresh Recipes cookbook. It has truly enabled me to take my healthy way of eating to the next level. Here are just some of the ways my Vitamix has changed my life:

- I am able to make whole food juices that do not discard the pulp.
- I can make my own fresh nut milk without any unnecessary ingredients and more cost effectively than buying cartons of it at the store.
- Unlimited combinations of smoothies can be made quickly and easily during my family's hectic morning rush.
- I can make and cook soup right in my Vitamix.
- I can chop vegetables and shred cabbage faster than I could by hand. By chopping just a little longer, I can make delicious chopped salads.
- I make my own hummus and nut butters so that I can control the ingredients used.

- I can use the dry grains container and prepare bread dough ready to pop in the oven.
- I whip up sorbets and non-dairy ice creams that my family can enjoy anytime of the day, and if you've ever purchased non-dairy ice cream, you know how expensive it is.

I couldn't ask for an easier clean-up afterward. Just a few drops of dish liquid in half a container of warm water blended for about 30 seconds is all that it takes to clean. Just rinse and air dry and you're ready to use it again!

I can save you $25 (United States customers) or $35 (Canadian customers) off of your shipping expense if you use the following promotional code when ordering either online at www.vitamix.com or by calling 1-800-848-2649. I do receive a small commission from Vitamix for every purchase made using my promotional code, but would highly recommend it even if I didn't.

Promotional Code 06-008273

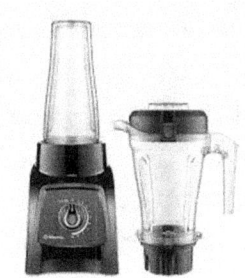

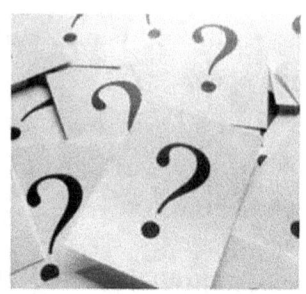

Commonly Asked Questions

Why should I consider making such a drastic change to my lifestyle? There is nothing wrong with me. Why should I fix something that isn't broken?

Let me share with you some advice from the experts in this field:

- "Do not confuse the absence of symptoms with the absence of disease." Pam Popper, ND
- "The first sign of heart disease 40% of the time is instant death." Pam Popper, ND
- "Stroke attacks with no warning signs, and results in death 25% of the time." Rip Esselstyn
- "In healthy people with no apparent diseases, it is estimated that they lose about 1/3 of their kidney function by the time they reach the age of 70 because of the high protein nature of the rich, American diet." John McDougall, MD
- "If you have vascular disease anywhere, you have it everywhere." Terry Mason, MD

Your body may be providing you with subtle clues that a dietary change is in order. Paying attention to these clues and making the appropriate changes now may help you to avoid a major health catastrophe later. Do you experience chest pain, indigestion, or heartburn on a regular basis? Have you had kidney or gallstones?

frequent constipation? pain in your legs when you walk? arthritic aches and pains? lack of energy? Do you just feel like you could feel better?

If the answer is yes to any of these questions, give yourself just 21 days to see how much better you can feel.

Where do I get my protein?

Only about 5-10% of your calories should come from protein. The health of highly developed civilizations such as the United States are often jeopardized by consuming an excess of protein. Osteoporosis and kidney stones are just two examples of diseases of affluence caused by consuming too much protein.

There is adequate but not excessive protein in a low-fat, plant-based lifestyle. The key to success is variety. Starches are a nutritionally complete food and pasta has a surprising amount of protein, about 10 grams in every 2 ounces. Plants are plentiful in protein containing anywhere from 6% to 28% of their calories in protein. Legumes are particularly protein-rich and vegetables contain a fair amount of protein as well. Broccoli has more protein as a percentage of its calories than steak!

Where do I get my fat?

Fat is an essential part of our diet and is responsible for the structure and maintenance of cells and hormones, healthy skin and hair, and the metabolism of fat-soluble vitamins. There are two essential fatty acids, essential because our bodies cannot synthesize them. We must obtain them from the food we eat. They are alpha-linolenic acid, an omega-3 fatty acid, and linoleic acid, an omega-6 fatty acid.

Most people in this country consume far too much fat and the fat that they consume is too heavily comprised of omega-6 fatty acids, largely due to the meat and dairy in their meals. We should strive for a balance in our intake of omega-3 and omega-6 fatty acids. This is easily accomplished by consuming plants. Omega-3 fatty acids are not as widespread as omega-6 fatty acids, so I recommend that you include one tablespoon of chia seed, hemp seed, ground flax seed, or walnuts daily.

The quality of flax oil varies greatly among brands and the oil itself is very fragile, so I suggest consuming ground flax seed in lieu of flax oil whenever possible.

Many people are under the assumption that fish oil is a good source of omega-3 fatty acids. While they do contain omega-3 fatty acids, only about 30% of their fat is omega-3. The remaining 70% is unhealthy, saturated fat. In addition, it is virtually impossible to find fish that have not been living in contaminated waters and if the fish is farmed, they may also contain antibiotic residues.

Vegetable oils, including the so-called healthful olive oil, are the strongest promoters of cancer that we commonly come into contact with and damage our arteries just as severely as animal fat.

Diets high in fat even change the viscosity or thickness of our blood. Instead of resembling water, our blood appears more like oil after eating a high-fat meal. This phenomenon is referred to as blood sludging.

If you experience painful menstrual cramps each month, adopting a low-fat, plant-based lifestyle may help to alleviate them. The higher the fat content in the food we eat, the higher our estrogen levels will rise during the month, and the farther they will have to fall at the end of our cycle, leading to more intense symptoms. The same holds true for menopausal symptoms. Lifetime exposure to elevated hormone levels as a result of eating a meat and dairy-centered diet could cause a more pronounced decrease of hormones at menopause, and lead to more severe symptoms.

No matter how hard we try, it is impossible to completely eliminate fat from our plate. There are trace amounts of healthy fat in whole grains, beans, vegetables, fruit, nuts, and seeds. These foods supply all the fat that our bodies need, about 3%-5% of our daily calories.

There are some plant foods that are higher in fat and should be eaten sparingly. Examples include nuts, nut butters, seeds, olives, avocados, coconut, and full-fat tofu.

I don't think something I'm eating is agreeing with me. My stools have not been normal. They're loosely formed lately. Should I stop eating this way?

For the first time in your life, your stools, in fact your bowel movements, may be exactly the way they should be. What is considered to be a normal bowel movement for a person eating the typical American diet is far from health promoting. In John McDougall, MD's book, Dr. McDougall's Digestive Tune-up, he has a chapter titled, "In Search of the Perfect Bowel Movement." What most people don't realize is that your activity, or inactivity, in the bathroom is a critical indicator of your gastrointestinal health and your risk for certain chronic, degenerative diseases.

According to Dr. McDougall, a perfect bowel movement includes feces that are soft and usually unformed, although they may be tubular. They will often break apart in the toilet bowl. The color of the stool can be anywhere from light yellow to brown, although certain plants will impart their colors on the stool, such as beets. The typical American diet, containing a large proportion of heme iron-laden meat, causes the typical American stool to be darker brown. It is perfectly normal to find undigested plant material in the stool. Bowel movements should last about 90 seconds from start to clean-up! Frequency of elimination is not as big a factor if you are moving your bowels with ease. If you are straining to defecate, changes need to be made to your dietary lifestyle. Straining is not an indicator of health.

Your bowels may be a bit overactive when you first start eating a low-fat, plant-based lifestyle, but should settle down into a more normal pattern within a couple of weeks. Meanwhile, you may want to spend the time finding a new place in your house for all of those books and magazines!

How long it takes for food to get from one end to the other can impact your cancer risk. Your stools flush out excess estrogen and cholesterol. If your transit time is 24-36 hrs, you are most likely meeting the half pound daily fecal output target for cancer prevention. If your transit time is 2 or more days, you are likely not meeting the target. A good bathroom scale can also help you to assess this. If you are not where you should be, increase consumption of the naturally occurring fiber in whole grains, legumes, vegetables, and fruits accompanied by 64 ounces of filtered water per day.

Does sugar feed cancer cells?

According to The Cancer Project (http://pcrm.org/health/cancer-resources/), no. White table sugar, corn syrup, and other highly processed, refined carbohydrates that contain additives and preservatives are not health foods, but do not "feed" cancer cells per se. They can, however, lead to obesity, which increases both diabetes and cancer risk.

Minimally processed whole grains, legumes, vegetables, and fruit eventually get broken down into glucose, however, they are in their natural form coupled with naturally occurring fiber, antioxidants and other phytochemicals, and are the body's preferred primary source of fuel.

Is soy safe to eat if I have cancer or if I'm a cancer survivor? Is soy safe for boys and men?

Per The Cancer Project (http://pcrm.org/health/cancer-resources/), "large human studies find whole soy foods such as tofu, tempeh, edamame, miso, and soy milk safe and healthy for women with a history of breast cancer. The general dietary recommendation from oncology dietitians and well-known cancer organizations promote up to three servings a day. Use of soy-based dietary supplements is not encouraged because researchers have not identified the safety of concentrated sources of soy for women with a dietary history of cancer. The bottom line: stick to food."

The Cancer Project provides the following analogy. Our cells contain estrogen receptors to which estrogens attach and are able to influence our cell's chemistry. The phytoestrogens that exist in soy act similar to a very weak form of our own estrogens. These receptor sites are like an airport jet way. When an airplane is attached to a jet way, no other airplanes can access that jet way. When the phytoestrogens in soy attach themselves to one of our estrogen receptor sites, it is as though a small, private jet has attached itself to the jet way. It prevents our own, more potent estrogens, a jumbo jet for example, from attaching to that very same jet way.

As with any plant food, variety and moderation are key. You should eat a variety of minimally processed, whole plant foods without overemphasizing any one food. The same can be said of whole soy products.

Soy protein isolate is an artificial food and should be given careful consideration before being included in a low-fat, plant-based lifestyle, especially if you have cancer. Please refer to the section in my book on soy protein isolate.

Soy phytoestrogens do not appear to have any adverse effects on male sexual development, fertility, or hormone levels.

Despite the fact that most people think of tofu when a plant-based lifestyle is mentioned, soy is not a required ingredient on the menu. If you prefer, a nutrient-dense, minimally processed, whole plant food lifestyle is easy to achieve and enjoy without any soy products at all.

Are there any additional strategies I can implement if I want to try to prevent cancer, if I have cancer, or if I'm a cancer survivor?

What you choose to eat and drink can have a powerful influence over this disease, however, in order to reduce cancer risk or significantly alter its course, dietary changes need to be significant. Be scrupulous about eliminating all animal products and added vegetable oils.

In addition, Michael Greger, MD, The Cancer Project, and John McDougall, MD also recommend the following:

- Beta-carotene's immune boosting effect can be seen by eating as few as two large cooked carrots per day. The beta-carotene is more readily available if the carrots are cooked. Studies have determined that beta-carotene found naturally in food is very cancer protective. However, beta-carotene when taken in isolated supplement form, was actually found to increase the incidence of lung cancer. Please get your nutrients from your food, with the exception of vitamin B_{12}, and vitamin D from sunshine.

- By eating one Brazil nut per day, you will provide yourself with vitamin E and selenium, two powerful components in your anti-cancer arsenal.

- Vitamin C is another powerful antioxidant. Include citrus fruits and vegetables such as raw red bell peppers, cooked Brussels sprouts, and raw broccoli on your plate often.

- Be very generous with the cruciferous vegetables that you eat. These include: arugula, bok choy, broccoli, Brussels sprouts, cabbage, cauliflower, collard greens, horseradish, kale, kohlrabi, mustard greens, radishes, rutabaga, turnip greens, turnips, and watercress.

- The sulforaphane produced when we eat broccoli, and especially broccoli sprouts, appears to inhibit breast cancer stem cells. Sulforaphane also appears to have anti-proliferative capabilities as well (suppressing the metastatic potential of cancer). If eating broccoli sprouts, aim for between ¼ and 1 ¼ cups each day. Both estrogen receptor positive and negative tumors were found to respond to sulforaphane. Michael Greger, MD has several poignant videos on the effect of certain foods on cancer. This is one of my favorite videos about the profound effect of broccoli on breast cancer:

http://pinterest.com/pin/225954106276238711/

- Sulforaphane, the active ingredient in broccoli and broccoli sprouts, may protect our brain, protect our eyesight, protect us from free radicals, induce our detoxification enzymes, help prevent cancer as well as help treat it, and can target breast cancer stem cells. The formation of this compound, however, requires the mixing of a precursor compound (glucoraphanin) with an enzyme (myrosinase) in broccoli. Myrosinase is destroyed by cooking. Therefore, Michael Greger, MD recommends the hack and hold technique. Chop cruciferous vegetables, wait 40 minutes, then they can be cooked and not lose their ability to create sulforaphane. Commercially produced frozen broccoli lacks the ability to form sulforaphane because the vegetables are blanched (flash cooked) before they are frozen for the very purpose of deactivating enzymes in order to extend shelf life in the frozen food section. However, adding myrosinase enzymes in the form of even a pinch of mustard powder, daikon radish, horseradish, wasabi, or a small amt of fresh greens to cooked cruciferous vegetables can offer anti-cancer sulforaphane levels comparable to raw, removing the necessity to pre-chop and eat raw for maximum health benefits.
- Eat often from the allium group of vegetables including: chives, garlic, green onions, leeks, onions, and shallots. Garlic is especially important. Make sure if you are cooking with garlic, that you let it sit for about ten minutes between being crushed and being cooked to maximize its beneficial effects.

- Lycopene, found in tomatoes, watermelon, and pink grapefruit, is another important component to your meals. Lycopene is more easily absorbed from tomatoes if they are cooked and even if they are in the form of spaghetti sauce, pizza sauce, and ketchup.

- Recent studies highlighted by Dr. Greger demonstrate the profound effect mushrooms can have on our cancer risk and our battle against cancer. Post-menopausal women naturally have lower estrogen levels than pre-menopausal women. Researchers have discovered that some breast cancer cells, perhaps as many as 70%, have developed the ability to synthesize their own estrogen out of testosterone with the help of the body's enzyme, aromatase. Plain, white mushrooms have been found to be the most effective at acting as an aromatase inhibitor to block breast tumor estrogen production. Just 5 white button mushrooms per day was found to be sufficient to suppress breast tumor growth. Those that ate ½ mushroom per day on average reduced their breast cancer risk by 64%. The same risk reduction occurs with dried mushrooms. In another study, the consumption of just a ½ teabag's worth of green tea per day along with ½ mushroom per day reduced breast cancer risk by nearly 90%. L-Ergothioneine, an essential amino acid, is cytoprotectant (protects cells). It gets into the nucleus of our cells to protect our DNA and into our mitochondria to act as a potent mitochondrial antioxidant. We only get it through our diet and cells don't do well when they are starved of it. It is made by microbes in the soil and is taken up by the root system of plants. It is widely distributed, but not evenly distributed, in both the plant and animal kingdoms. Fungus (mushrooms) have nearly 40 times more than its closest competitor, beans. Here is just one of the videos Dr. Greger has on the powerful effect of mushrooms on cancer:

- Eat berries and dark, green, leafy vegetables as often as possible. Eat beets and apple peels regularly.

- Flax seed is incredibly powerful at dampening the effects of estrogen. Just one tablespoon per day can extend a woman's menstrual cycle by approximately one day per month on average, resulting in fewer periods throughout her lifetime. The resulting lower lifetime estrogen exposure can equate to lower breast cancer risk. Frequent bladder infections can increase breast cancer risk as the antibiotics used to treat them wipe out the beneficial gut flora that take flax seed lignans and turn them into anti-cancer compounds.

- Cranberries and lemons can cause a dramatic drop in cancer cell proliferation just being consumed in tiny doses.

- Soy intake during any stage of life decreases breast cancer risk but the strongest risk reduction occurs when soy intake begins during childhood. It can cut later risk of breast cancer by as much as half. It can also sensitize us to the protective effects of soy consumption in adulthood. If soy consumption begins during adolescence or adulthood, the risk reduction is about 25%. Soy's phytoestrogens have been found to be protective against cancer, especially breast cancer, but too much soy can act like animal proteins in raising IGF-1 levels in our bloodstream due to soy's relative similarity to our own amino acid ratios. Current research recommends no more than 3-5 servings of soy per day.

- Spices like cloves (sprinkle on your oatmeal and sweet potatoes), dried peppermint (sprinkle on salads, focaccia, tabouleh, and Indian food), dried lemon balm (makes a nice tea), allspice, marjoram (sprinkle on pasta), cinnamon (sprinkle on oatmeal and sweet potatoes), oregano (sprinkle on pasta), and turmeric/pepper together all have potent antioxidant properties.

- The spice turmeric has an anti-proliferative cancer effect. It is actually being considered for use with multi-drug resistant breast cancer. However, keep consumption to less than 1 teaspoon per day due to its oxalate content and potential to create oxalate kidney stones.

- Add 1 teaspoon amla powder (dried Indian gooseberries found in Indian grocery stores) to your favorite smoothie recipe for a potent antioxidant boost.

- Water is critical to good health. By adding two simple ingredients to your water, you can consume what Michael Greger, MD describes as possibly the highest antioxidant beverage in the world, hibiscus/lemon water. The recipe is located in the beverage suggestion in the What is a Plant-Based Lifestyle? chapter.

- In another study, Dr. Greger found that regular green tea drinkers reduce their breast cancer risk by about 1/3 compared to those that do not regularly drink green tea.

- Reconsider your alcohol intake. Even one drink per day, if consumed every day, increases breast cancer risk. Alcohol consumption can also increase the risk of liver and colorectal cancer.

- Avoid products which contain soy protein isolate. Studies have demonstrated that consumption of 40 grams of soy protein isolate daily can increase your cancer risk.

- As I mentioned earlier, how long it takes for food to get from one end to the other can impact your cancer risk. Your stools flush out excess estrogen and cholesterol. If your transit time is 24-36 hrs, you are most likely meeting the half pound daily fecal output target for cancer prevention. If your transit time is 2 or more days, you are likely not meeting the target. A good bathroom scale can also help you to assess this. If you are not where you should be, increase consumption of the naturally occurring fiber in whole grains, legumes, vegetables, and fruits accompanied by 64 ounces of filtered water per day.

- Exercise helps to protect against cancer by stimulating natural killer (NK) cell activity. NK cells work to eliminate tumor cells as well as virus-infected cells.

- Get 10-15 minutes of sunshine on your face, neck, chest, and arms between 10 am and 2 pm daily as often as you can (without sunscreen). If you burn, reduce the time slightly until you don't burn. This is the best way to get your vitamin D, which is very cancer protective. The vitamin D you acquire in the spring, summer, and fall should cover your needs through the winter.

Do I have to buy all organic? What if that isn't possible?

Buy organic when you can. If it is too expensive or if the quality of the organic produce is poor, The Environmental Working Group makes recommendations each year as to the produce that should be purchased organic whenever possible, The Dirty Dozen, and the produce of which you need to worry less, The Clean Fifteen. Here is the link:

http://www.ewg.org/foodnews/summary/

Recipes

Warning for those with advanced heart disease, cancer, or an autoimmune disorder: It is imperative that you do not consume added oils including vegetable oils. Any recipes that call for oil will either need to be avoided or adapted to remove any added oils.

Breakfast

Oatmeal

Old fashioned oatmeal cooked with filtered water or non-dairy milk with any or all of the following ingredients:

- o fresh, frozen, or dried fruit
- o 100% fruit spread
- o cinnamon
- o pure vanilla extract
- o nuts and/or seeds
- o topped with 1 tablespoon chia seed, hemp seed, or ground flax seed
- o wheat germ

The Ultimate Smoothie
From Tracey Eakin
www.youtube.com/watch?v=0HdkFeBstnw

Makes 4 1-cup servings

1 container of blueberry non-dairy yogurt
1 container of strawberry non-dairy yogurt
2 tablespoons of freshly ground flax seeds (I dedicate a coffee grinder
     for the grinding of my flax seeds.)
2 tablespoons of wheat germ
2 tablespoons of shelled hemp seeds (optional)
2 teaspoons maca (optional)
1/3 cup coarsely chopped raw walnuts
4 coarsely chopped raw Brazil nuts
2/3 cup unsweetened coconut milk or other non-dairy milk
1 banana
1 cup frozen, organic mixed berries (strawberries, blueberries, raspber
     ries, and blackberries)
2 tablespoons of Vitamineral Green (an intense and comprehensive
     array of nature's most nutritive and cleansing super foods
     grown and processed in a manner in which they retain their
     potency) (optional, can use fresh dark, leafy greens instead)

Place all ingredients in a large bowl and blend with a stick blender or
place all ingredients in a traditional blender and mix well.

307 calories and 10 grams of protein per serving

Michael Greger, MD's Smoothie
http://nutritionfacts.org/video/a-better-breakfast/

1 cup unsweetened soy milk
½ cup frozen blueberries
pulp of ripe, Mexican mango
1 tablespoon ground flax seed
palmful of bulk white tea leaves
1 teaspoon amla powder (available at Indian grocery stores)
handful of sprouted lentils

Blend all ingredients and enjoy.

It's Easy Being Green Smoothie
By Chef AJ

16 ounces of freshly squeezed orange juice (or 2-3 fresh oranges)
1 bunch kale (approximately 12 ounces)
2 frozen, ripe bananas
2 cups frozen mango
fresh mint leaves to taste (optional)

In a blender, blend orange juice (or oranges) with kale until smooth. Add frozen fruit and blend until completely blended and thick.

For a Creamsicle effect, use half unsweetened almond milk and half orange juice. You can also use spinach instead of kale.

Michael Greger, MD's Pumpkin Pie Smoothie

http://nutritionfacts.org/video/spicing-up-dna-protection/?utm_source=rss&utm_medium=rss&utm_campaign=spicing-up-dna-protection&utm_source=NutritionFacts.org&utm_campaign=91c3d9eb50-RSS_VIDEO_DAILY&utm_medium=email&utm_term=0_40f9e497d1-91c3d9eb50-21951209

1 can of pumpkin
frozen cranberries
pitted dates
pumpkin pie spice
non-dairy milk
turmeric

Blend and enjoy.

Spelt-Blueberry Pancakes
From Engine 2 Diet

2 cups spelt flour
2 cups oat flour (Finely grind old fashioned oats in a food processor.)
2 tablespoons baking powder (Choose non-aluminum.)
4 tablespoons ground flax seed
½ teaspoon salt
3 ½ cups non-dairy milk
4 tablespoons unsweetened applesauce
2 tablespoons agave nectar (I use pure maple syrup.)
1 tablespoon pure vanilla extract
2 cups blueberries (I use frozen blueberries and it turns out fine.)

Whisk the flours, baking powder, ground flax seed, and salt together in a large bowl. Combine the wet ingredients in another bowl.

Form a well in the center of the dry ingredients and add wet ingredients. Stir the batter just until the dry ingredients are thoroughly moistened. It will seem very thin, but will thicken.

Let the batter rest for 15 minutes (spelt flour takes a little longer to absorb liquids). If you can't wait, your pancakes won't be as crisp.

After the batter has rested, fold in blueberries.

Heat a dry skillet until a drop of water dances on its surface. Immediately prior to pouring the pancake batter onto the hot skillet, sprinkle a very light dusting of spelt flour onto the surface of the skillet. This will help to prevent your pancakes from sticking to the surface.

Cook until the batter begins to bubble and the bottom of the pancake is golden brown. Flip and cook the other side.

Tofu French Toast
From The Cancer Survivor's Guide by Neal D. Barnard, MD and Jennifer K. Reilly, RD

Makes 6 1-slice servings.

8 ounces low-fat silken tofu
1 ripe banana
½ cup water (I like to use non-dairy milk.)
1 teaspoon light molasses or pure maple syrup (I like to use pure maple
     syrup.)
½ teaspoon ground cinnamon
½ teaspoon pure vanilla extract (not in the original recipe, but I like to
add it)
6 slices whole wheat bread

Combine the tofu, banana, water (or non-dairy milk), molasses (or pure maple syrup), cinnamon, and vanilla in a blender and process until smooth. Pour into a shallow dish.

Place a nonstick skillet over medium heat. Dip each slice of bread (both sides) into the banana mixture and brown it on both sides in the skillet. You will need to brown the bread in several batches depending on the size of your skillet.

Stored in a covered container in the refrigerator, leftover Tofu French Toast will keep for up to 2 days.

Per serving: 123 calories; 2.9 g fat; 0.5 g saturated fat; 21.4% calories from fat; 0 mg cholesterol; 6.1 g protein; 20.4 g carbohydrate; 6.1 g sugar; 3.6 g fiber; 151 mg sodium; 46 mg calcium; 2.1 mg iron; 2.1 mg vitamin C; 7 mcg beta-carotene; 0.2 mg vitamin E

Apple-Maple Fusion Topping
From Jo Stepaniak

Pure maple syrup is unquestionably delicious, but it's also high in calories and a bit expensive. To reduce the cost to your waistline and your wallet, try this fabulous blend. It is so easy to make, adds a bit of extra nutrition, and extends the maple syrup while retaining all of its magnificent flavor. It's the perfect topping for pancakes, waffles, or French toast.

Makes about 1 cup

½ cup pure maple syrup
½ cup unsweetened applesauce

Stir together maple syrup and applesauce until well blended. Serve at room temperature, or warm briefly over low heat. Store leftovers in the refrigerator.

Healthy Hash Brown Casserole
From Susan Voisin, FatFree Vegan Kitchen
http://blog.fatfreevegan.com/2013/02/healthy-hash-brown-casserole.html

Susan has asked that her recipes not be re-posted. Please follow the link above for the recipe.

Home Fries, Braised Mixed Vegetables, Toast, and Fruit
From Tracey Eakin

This is now my family's favorite Saturday morning breakfast. Missing from the picture are whole grain toast and fruit.

I keep the skins on the potatoes and begin cooking the slices in the microwave until soft. This speeds up cooking time in the skillet. While the potatoes are cooking in the microwave, I sauté chopped onions, minced garlic, chopped green peppers, and chopped celery (because those are the vegetables my children will eat right now) in a little bit of water until the onions are translucent and the peppers are soft. Once the potatoes are soft, I add ½ tablespoon olive oil for as many potatoes as will fit my largest skillet and finish the potatoes by browning them in the skillet. I add salt and pepper to taste.

I braise the rest of the vegetables separately and as each additional vegetable is accepted by my children, I add it into the main skillet. In this picture, I braised shredded purple cabbage, chopped red bell peppers, and chopped asparagus in a little water until soft. I continue to add small amounts of water as needed to keep the vegetables from sticking and add salt and pepper to taste. For a little heat, I add a pinch of cayenne pepper or a small amount of crushed red pepper flakes. I like to be adventurous and rotate the vegetables that I use. I challenge myself to keep trying to find additional vegetables to include. Missing from the picture are one of my favorites, mushrooms.

gRAWnola
From Chef AJ

4 pounds old-fashioned oats
5 cups date paste (see recipe below)
1 ½ cups almond meal
1 tablespoon roasted cinnamon
½ tablespoon cardamom
2 pounds raisins

Using food service gloves, mix all ingredients together except for the raisins until date paste is evenly distributed. Place the mixture on dehydrator trays fitted with Teflex sheets and dehydrate for 24-48 hours until desired crunchiness is reached. Stir in the raisins. Keep in an airtight container.

Date Paste
From Chef AJ

Make sure you always have some on hand to create a healthy dessert in no time.

1 pound pitted dates
1 cup liquid (water, unsweetened non-dairy milk, unsweetened juice)

Soak dates in liquid overnight or for several hours until much of the liquid is absorbed. In a food processor fitted with the "S" blade, process dates and liquid until completely smooth. Store date paste in the refrigerator.

Better-Than-Boxed Strawberry and Oat Breakfast Cereal
From YumUniverse,
http://www.yumuniverse.com/2012/05/24/better-than-boxed-strawberry-oat-breakfast-cereal/

Buckwheat and Oat Bites (optional but worth including):
1 cup oat flour
¼ cup buckwheat flour
¼ cup brown rice flour (if you don't have any, use 1/4 cup more oat
    flour)
1 teaspoon aluminum-free baking powder
¼ cup Sucanat (available at health food stores)
¼ teaspoon sea salt
2 teaspoons fresh lemon juice
1 tablespoon unrefined, cold-pressed coconut oil, warmed to liquid
½ teaspoon vanilla extract
2 tablespoons chia seeds
1 cup warm water

1 cup dried strawberries (Any dried fruit will work.)

Cereal Ingredients:
2 cups oatmeal
1 cup chopped walnuts
1 cup chopped almonds
½ cup hulled sunflower seeds
¼ cup sesame seeds (I used roasted sesame seeds and it added addi
    tional flavor.)
¼ cup chia seeds
½ cup pure maple syrup
1 tablespoon unrefined, cold-pressed coconut oil
2 tablespoons Sucanat
½ teaspoon sea salt

Preheat oven to 350 degrees F.

In a glass mixing bowl, sift together oat flour, buckwheat flour, brown rice flour, baking powder, Sucanat, and sea salt.

In another glass bowl, whisk together the lemon juice, coconut oil, vanilla, chia seeds, and water.

Fold together with silicone spatula.

Drop individual dollops of batter onto two parchment-lined cookie sheets from a pastry bag or from a plastic freezer bag with a tiny corner cut off of it after it has been filled with the batter.

Bake for 15 minutes. Remove from oven and allow to cool.

In a large bowl, place all of the cereal ingredients and fold together. Do not include the buckwheat and oat bites or dried strawberries.

Spread onto a parchment-lined cookie sheet and bake for 20 minutes at the same temperature, 350 degrees F.

Allow to cool entirely. Mix together with buckwheat and oat bites and dried strawberries.

Fill a small bowl, add some non-dairy milk, and enjoy!

Sprinkle freshly ground flax or hemp seeds on before eating for extra nutrition but remember to keep these seeds in the refrigerator until you are ready to eat. The essential fats are delicate and need to stay chilled and away from light.

Store in an airtight glass container or in a sealable plastic bag in the refrigerator.

Variations:
- Make the cereal without any dried fruit and try with different fresh fruit. Try bananas, mangoes, peaches, blueberries, blackberries, or raspberries.
- Try sprinkling with cardamom or cinnamon.
- Add 1 teaspoon cinnamon to the buckwheat and oat bites and another teaspoon to the cereal.
- When making the buckwheat and oat bites, boil the water and steep with organic, chamomile tea first.

- Add 1 teaspoon cardamom to buckwheat and oat bites and add 2 tablespoons cocoa powder to the cereal mixture. After the baked cereal cools completely, add vegan chocolate chips.

Maple-Cinnamon Peanut Butter Banana Toast
From Kathy Patalsky

http://kblog.lunchboxbunch.com/2013/07/maple-cinnamon-peanut-butter-
banana.html?utm_source=feedburner&utm_medium=email&utm_campaign=Feed%3A+KathysBlogHealthyHappyLife+%28Kathy%27s+Blog%3A+Healthy.+Happy.+Life.%29

Serves 1-2

2 slices whole grain bread
1 teaspoon and 1 tablespoon nut butter
1 ripe banana (bananas that are black-spotted work the best)
½ teaspoon maple syrup or agave nectar (optional)
1-2 pinches cinnamon

Possible toppings: shaved dark chocolate, seeds, a few raw, jungle peanuts, or more fruit

Mash the banana, 1 teaspoon nut butter, maple syrup, and cinnamon in a bowl. Toast bread and spread with 1 tablespoon nut butter. Top with the banana mash. Sprinkle with the toppings.

Scrambled Tofu
From Tracey Eakin

Scrambled tofu is a favorite for breakfast in my home. Even though it is often suggested as a replacement for scrambled eggs, it really is a completely different dish and shouldn't be judged in comparison to the taste and texture of scrambled eggs.

Apparently, black salt provides an egg-like flavor. I haven't tried this yet, but if you are making scrambled tofu in place of scrambled eggs, try sprinkling a little black salt on it to see if it makes it taste a little like scrambled eggs.

1 14-ounce container of low-fat, firm tofu
½ to 1/3 cup nutritional yeast depending upon taste
¼ teaspoon turmeric
¼ teaspoon black pepper or more to taste

Rinse block of tofu with water and crumble into non-stick frying pan. Heat on medium heat. Add enough water, about ¼ cup, to keep the tofu from sticking. Add more water as needed. Add turmeric and black pepper and stir to combine. Heat until hot.

Sometimes I sauté onion, minced garlic, bell peppers, mushrooms, and spinach in a small amount of water and add it to the scrambled tofu mixture. My children like to add roasted sesame seeds.

Vegan Blueberry Muffins with Crumb Topping
From http://www.vegancoach.com/vegan-breakfast.html#anchor-blueberry-muffins

Children love this recipe!

Makes 6 giant muffins or 12 small muffins.

paper muffin cups
1 ½ cups flour (best with half whole wheat and half unbleached white)
¾ cup Sucanat or other granulated sugar (I just use regular sugar.)
½ teaspoon sea salt
2 teaspoons aluminum-free baking powder
1/3 cup applesauce
1 tablespoon flax seeds
1/3 cup non-dairy milk (and extra non-dairy milk or orange juice as
        needed)
1 cup blueberries, fresh or defrosted frozen
¼ cup Sucanat or other granulated sugar (I just use regular sugar.)
1/8 cup whole wheat flour
1 tablespoon non-dairy butter (I recommend Earth Balance organic
buttery spread.)
¾ teaspoon cinnamon

Prepare a "flax egg". Grind 1 tablespoon flax seeds in a blender or food processor (I've only ever used a dedicated coffee grinder to grind flax seeds.). Slowly add 1/6 cup water and blend until it produces a gooey mixture (I transfer my flax seeds from my coffee grinder to a plastic bowl and blend the water into the seeds using a hand mixer.). Be sure to clean out the blender, food processor, or hand mixer immediately.

Preheat oven to 400 degrees F. Place paper muffin cups in muffin tins. Use unbleached baking cups if possible. Here is where you can buy them:
http://www.amazon.com/gp/product/B000E8X118/ref=s9_psimh_g w_p79_d0_i1?pf_rd_m=ATVPDKIKX0DER&pf_rd_s=center-2&pf_rd_r=0JKSJBGDJSE7VHX83ABM&pf_rd_t=101&pf_rd_p=1 630083502&pf_rd_i=507846

Combine flour, sugar, salt, and baking powder. Pour the applesauce into a 1 cup measuring cup, then add the flax egg and enough milk to fill the measuring cup. Add to dry ingredients and mix well. If batter is too dry, add more milk or some orange juice to moisten. Fold in blueberries, then place the batter into the muffin cups.

Mix ¼ cup Sucanat or other granulated sugar, 1/8 cup whole wheat flour, 1 tablespoon non-dairy butter, and ¾ teaspoon cinnamon until any large clumps are worked out. Sprinkle topping over muffin batter before baking.

Bake 15-20 minutes, until the topping and the tops of the muffins are golden. Allow to cool briefly on a wire rack before removing from muffin pan.

139 calories per 1 of 12 small muffins.

Spring Fling Scones
From Kathy Patalsky
http://kblog.lunchboxbunch.com/2014/03/spring-fling-scones.html

Makes 8 large scones.

Scone Ingredients:

2 cups white flour, organic
1 cup sugar, organic
12 ounces of silken tofu
2 tablespoons of flax seeds, ground
1 tablespoon chia seeds
2 tablespoons fresh orange juice and a pinch of orange zest
3 tablespoons extra virgin coconut oil, melted
1 tablespoon baking powder
1 teaspoon salt

Coloring:

2 tablespoons matcha green tea, culinary
1 tablespoon beets, grated or raspberries
½ teaspoon turmeric

Lemon-Vanilla Glaze:

1-2 drops vanilla extract
1 cup powdered sugar, organic
1 ½ tablespoons lemon juice
1 tablespoon coconut oil, melted

Directions:

Preheat oven to 400 degrees F.

Combine the flour, baking powder, salt, and sugar in a large mixing bowl.

In a blender on low speed, combine the silken tofu, orange juice, orange zest, chia seeds, coconut oil, and ground flax seed. Blend until smooth and thickened, about 1-2 minutes.

Fold the liquid mixture into the dry bowl until a fluffy dough forms.

Split the dough into thirds, transferring one third to a small bowl and another third to another small bowl.

In the large mixing bowl, fold the matcha into one third of the dough. Add a bit of flour if needed to handle. Knead until the matcha distributes creating a green color. It can be a bit swirled.

On a floured surface, press out the green dough into a round about 7-8 inches across. Form round with your hands. Again, a pinch more flour if things get sticky. Also, it helps to have your kitchen at a cool temperature so the oil-infused dough doesn't get too melty in texture.

Repeat the coloring steps with the yellow (using the turmeric) and pink (using the beets or raspberries) thirds of the dough. Place each layer on top of the green in a stacking form so that you end up with one fluffy round of dough, three layers of color. Using your hands, pat out and form the dough into a tall, fluffy round.

Using a chilled or lightly oiled knife, cut out the scones by slicing the dough in half, then in quarters, then again in eighths, just like pizza slices.

Place the scones on a lightly greased baking sheet (I used parchment paper instead and they turned out fine.) and place in the oven to bake for 20-25 minutes, or until the edges begin to brown just a tad and the tops are firm and toasty to touch. The scones will still be quite tender and fluffy on the inside and will need a few minutes to cool before pouring the glaze.

Cool scones on a baking rack. Whisk together the vanilla-lemon glaze. Pour the glaze over top of the scones after they have cooled a bit. Serve scones warm for best texture and flavor. Store in the freezer or refrigerator and warm up to serve.

I forgot to use the zest in preparing the wet ingredients for the scones, so I mixed it up in the glaze. It tasted wonderful and created beautiful orange specks in the lemon-vanilla glaze.

Lunch/Dinner Entrees and Side Dishes

Salads

Fruit and Vegetable Salad

Romaine lettuce
mandarin oranges
sliced strawberries or halved grapes
toasted walnuts
blueberries or raspberries
raspberry vinaigrette dressing

Hot Skillet Salad
From Susan Voisin, FatFree Vegan Kitchen
http://blog.fatfreevegan.com/2011/02/hot-skillet-salad.html

Susan has asked that her recipes not be re-posted. Please follow the link above for the recipe.

Potato Salad
From The Cancer Survivor's Guide by Neal D. Barnard, MD and Jennifer K. Reilly, RD

Makes about 4 1-cup servings.

2 medium potatoes, peeled and cut into 0.5" cubes for about 2.5 cups
     (I prefer not to peel them.)
½ cup diced sweet onion
½ cup diced celery
½ small red bell pepper, finely diced
¼ cup minced fresh parsley
1 teaspoon dried dill weed
¼ cup fat-free or low-fat vegan mayonnaise (I recommend Follow
     Your Heart Original Vegenaise Dressing & Sandwich Spread.)
1 tablespoon seasoned rice vinegar
1 ½ teaspoons mustard
1/8 teaspoon salt
1/8 teaspoon ground black pepper

Steam the potatoes until just barely tender when pierced with a knife, about 10 minutes. Do not overcook. Transfer to a large bowl and add the onion, celery, bell pepper, parsley, and dill weed.

In a separate bowl, combine the mayonnaise, vinegar, mustard, salt, and pepper. Mix well. Add to the potato mixture and toss gently until evenly distributed. Chill thoroughly before serving.

Stored in a covered container in the refrigerator, leftover potato salad will keep for up to 3 days.

Per serving: 135 calories; 3.8 g fat; 0.5 g saturated fat; 25.1% of calories from fat; 0 mg cholesterol; 2.9 g protein; 23.7 g carbohydrate; 4.7 g sugar; 3.4 g fiber; 289 mg sodium; 46 mg calcium; 2.3 mg iron; 36.4 mg vitamin C; 394 mcg beta-carotene; 1.1 mg vitamin E

Couscous Confetti Salad
From Physicians Committee for Responsible Medicine's 21-Day Vegan Kick Start Program
www.youtube.com/watch?v=ayE8LWLa0i4

Makes about 8 1-cup servings.

1 ½ cups dry whole wheat couscous (I prefer to use quinoa, pictured
      above.)
2 cups boiling water
3-4 green onions, finely chopped, including tops
1 red bell pepper, seeded and finely diced
1 carrot, grated
1-2 cups finely shredded red cabbage
½ cup finely chopped fresh parsley
½ cup golden raisins or chopped dried apricots
the juice of 1 lemon
¼ cup seasoned rice vinegar
1 tablespoon olive oil
1 teaspoon curry powder
1 ½ teaspoons salt

In a large bowl, combine couscous and boiling water. Stir to mix, then cover and let stand until all the water has been absorbed, 5-10 minutes. Fluff with a fork.

Add green onions, bell pepper, carrot, cabbage, parsley, and raisins or apricots.

In a small bowl, mix lemon juice, vinegar, oil, curry powder, and salt. Add to salad and toss to mix. Serve at room temperature or chilled.

Three Bean Salad
From Dreena Burton's Plant-Powered Kitchen

Serves 6 as a side dish.

4 cups combination of garbanzo beans, kidney beans, and black beans (rinse and drain first if using canned)
½ - ¾ cup green or red bell pepper, chopped (I use a colorful combination of red, yellow, and orange bell peppers.)
¼ cup celery, finely chopped
½ cup green onions (mostly green portion, not as much white), sliced
3 ½ tablespoons apple cider vinegar
1 tablespoon extra-virgin olive oil (keeps salad moist but is totally optional - omit for oil-free version) (I omit the oil and it still tastes great.)
½ - 1 tablespoon pure maple syrup
½ teaspoon Dijon mustard
½ teaspoon + 1/8 teaspoon sea salt
freshly ground black pepper, to taste
½ cup apple, chopped and tossed in ½ teaspoon lemon juice
couple pinches ground cloves

In a large bowl, combine all the ingredients (no need to mix the vinaigrette separately), tossing well to fully mix. Season to taste with extra salt and pepper if desired.

This salad tastes better after it's had about a day to sit and the beans have absorbed some of the marinade. Be sure to toss again prior to serving to redistribute any dressing lingering at the bottom of your container.

Corn and Black Bean Salad
www.youtube.com/watch?v=bLV-BQ0udFM

Preparation time: 10 minutes
Makes 4 servings

¼ cup balsamic vinegar
2 tablespoons olive oil (I eliminate the oil and it tastes just fine.)
½ teaspoon salt
½ teaspoon white sugar
½ teaspoon ground black pepper
½ teaspoon ground cumin
½ teaspoon chili powder
3 tablespoons chopped fresh cilantro
½ to 1 cup grape tomatoes or chopped tomatoes
1 15-ounce can black beans, rinsed and drained
1 8.75-ounce can sweet corn, drained

Mix balsamic vinegar, oil, salt, sugar, black pepper, cumin, and chili powder.

In a medium bowl, stir together grape tomatoes (if using chopped tomatoes, wait until just before serving to add), black beans, and corn. Toss with dressing and garnish with cilantro. Cover and refrigerate overnight.

Mexican Corn Salad
From Foods that Fight Pain by Neal D. Barnard, MD

Makes 6 servings

1 15-ounce can corn, drained
1 large cucumber, peeled and diced
½ cup finely chopped red onion
1 medium red bell pepper, seeded and finely diced
1 medium tomato, seeded and diced
½ cup chopped fresh cilantro
2 tablespoons seasoned rice vinegar
2 tablespoons cider vinegar or distilled vinegar
1 tablespoon lemon or lime juice (I prefer lemon juice.)
1 garlic clove, minced
1 teaspoon ground cumin
1 teaspoon ground coriander
1/8 teaspoon cayenne pepper

In a large salad bowl, combine corn, cucumber, onion, bell pepper, tomato, and cilantro, if using. In a small bowl, combine vinegars, lemon or lime juice, garlic, cumin, coriander, and cayenne. Pour over the salad and toss gently to mix.

Per serving (1/6 of the recipe): 71 calories; 0.8 g fat; 0.1 g saturated fat; 10.3% calories from fat; 0 mg cholesterol; 2.2 g protein; 15.8 g carbohydrate; 6.2 g sugar; 2.4 g fiber; 188 mg sodium; 22 mg calcium; 1 mg iron; 47.7 mg vitamin C; 455 mcg beta-carotene; 0.5 mg vitamin E

Hoppin' John Salad
From The Cancer Survivor's Guide by Neal D. Barnard, MD and Jennifer K. Reilly, RD

1 ½ cups cooked or canned black-eyed peas, rinsed and drained
1 ½ cups cooked brown rice
1 tomato, diced
½ cup thinly sliced green onions
½ cup thinly sliced celery
2 tablespoons minced fresh parsley
¼ cup freshly squeezed lemon juice
1 tablespoon olive oil
1-2 garlic cloves, minced or pressed
¼ teaspoon salt

Combine the black-eyed peas, rice, tomato, green onions, celery, and parsley in a mixing bowl.

Whisk together the lemon juice, oil, garlic, and salt in a small bowl. Pour over the salad and toss gently until evenly distributed. If time permits, chill for 1-2 hours before serving to allow the flavors to blend.

Stored in a covered container in the refrigerator, leftover Hoppin' John Salad will keep for up to three days.

Per serving: 91 calories; 1.9 g fat; 0.3 g saturated fat; 18.5% calories from fat; 0 mg cholesterol; 3.7 g protein; 15.4 g carbohydrate; 1.3 g sugar; 3.6 g fiber; 68 mg sodium; 20 mg calcium; 1.2 mg iron; 5.4 mg vitamin C; 137 mcg beta-carotene; 0.4 mg vitamin E

Marinated Lentil Salad
From Ecological Cooking: Recipes to Save the Planet

Makes 4-6 servings.

Salad:

1 cup green lentils
4 cups water
1 cup grated carrots
½ cup red onions, finely chopped
½ cup minced fresh parsley
1 clove garlic, pressed

Dressing:

1 tablespoon oil
2 tablespoons balsamic vinegar
1 tablespoon Dijon mustard
1 teaspoon oregano
1 teaspoon vegan Worcestershire sauce
½ teaspoon salt (optional)
¼ teaspoon freshly ground black pepper

Cook the lentils in the water for 30 minutes, until tender but still firm. Drain. Place in a mixing bowl along with the remaining salad ingredients. In a separate bowl, whisk together the dressing ingredients. Pour over the lentils and toss to mix. Chill several hours before serving, to allow flavors to blend.

French Lentil Salad
From Skinny Bitch in the Kitch by Rory Freedman and Kim Barnouin

Serves 6 to 8.

1 cup French green lentils (Any lentils work just fine.)
2 cups water
6 tablespoons extra virgin olive oil (I use 3 tablespoons and it turns out
     just fine.)
2 tablespoons white wine vinegar or champagne vinegar
½ tablespoon fresh chopped or 0.5 teaspoon dry tarragon
1 teaspoon Dijon mustard
1 teaspoon fine sea salt
½ teaspoon pepper
2 tomatoes, cut into ½ - inch dice
2 large Belgian endive (about 8 ounces), halved lengthwise and cut into
½ - inch slices (Can use regular   endive.)
1 green bell pepper, cut into ½ - inch dice
1 yellow bell pepper, cut into ½ - inch dice
½ cup chopped fresh Italian parsley

In a 1- to 2-quart saucepan over high, combine the lentils and water and bring to a boil. Reduce the heat to a simmer, cover, and cook 35 to 45 minutes, until the lentils are al dente, tender but not mushy.

Meanwhile, in a small bowl, whisk together the olive oil, vinegar, tarragon, mustard, salt, and pepper.

Once the lentils are cooked, drain any water left in the pot and transfer the lentils to a large bowl. Toss with about half the dressing and set aside to cool to room temperature.

Once the lentils are cool, stir in the tomatoes, endive, bell peppers, and parsley. Add the remaining dressing, tossing gently. Serve cold or at room temperature.

Marinated Zucchini and Chickpea Salad
From Susan Voisin, FatFree Vegan Kitchen
http://blog.fatfreevegan.com/2013/07/marinated-zucchini-and-chickpea-salad.html

Susan has asked that her recipes not be re-posted. Please follow the link above for the recipe.

Soups and Stews

Black Bean and Salsa Soup
From Annie's Eats
http://www.annies-eats.com/2007/10/14/black-bean-and-salsa-soup/

Keep the ingredients in your pantry for when you have absolutely no time to make something for lunch or dinner.

Serves about 4

2 cans black beans, drained and rinsed
1 ½ cups vegetable broth
1 cup salsa
1 teaspoon cumin
salt and pepper to taste
vegan sour cream
green onions

Combine beans, broth, salsa, and cumin in a blender. Blend until fairly smooth. Season with salt and pepper to taste. Heat in either a sauce pan or in the microwave until thoroughly heated. Put in soup bowls and garnish with a dollop of vegan sour cream and chopped green onions.

Summer Minestrone
From Fields of Greens: New Vegetarian Recipes from the
Celebrated Greens Restaurant by Annie Somerville

Makes 8 to 9 cups.

½ cup dried red beans, about 3 ounces, sorted and soaked overnight
6 cups cold water
2 bay leaves
2 fresh sage leaves (I use ¼ teaspoon ground sage)
1 fresh oregano sprig (I use ½ teaspoon dried oregano)
1 tablespoon extra virgin olive oil
1 medium-sized red onion, diced, about 2 cups
salt and pepper
¼ teaspoon dried basil
¼ teaspoon dried oregano
6 garlic cloves, finely chopped
1 small carrot, diced, about ¾ cup
1 small red bell pepper, diced, about ¾ cup
1 small zucchini, diced, about ¾ cup
¼ cup dry red wine
2 pounds fresh tomatoes, peeled, seeded, and coarsely chopped, about
        3 cups, or 1 28-ounce can tomatoes with juice, coarsely
        chopped
¼ cup small pasta, cooked al dente, drained, and rinsed
1/3 bunch fresh spinach or chard, cut into thin ribbons and washed,
        about 2 cups packed
2 tablespoons chopped fresh basil

Drain and rinse the beans. Place them in a 2-quart saucepan with the
water, 1 bay leaf, the sage leaves, and the oregano. Bring to a boil,
reduce the heat, and simmer, uncovered, until the beans are tender,
about 30 minutes. Remove the herbs.

While the beans are cooking, heat the olive oil in a soup pot. Add the
onion, ½ teaspoon salt, the dried herbs, and a few pinches of pepper.
Sauté the onion over medium heat until soft, 5 to 7 minutes. Add the
garlic, carrots, peppers, and zucchini and sauté for 7 to 8 minutes. Add
the wine and cook for 1 or 2 minutes, until the pan is almost dry. Add

the tomatoes, 1 teaspoon salt, 1/8 teaspoon pepper, and the remaining bay leaf. Simmer for 15 minutes, then add the pasta, spinach or chard, and beans with their broth. Season with salt and pepper to taste. Add the fresh basil just before serving.

I added an extra cup of water toward the end and let it simmer in.

Red Bean, Potato, and Arugula Soup
From Moosewood Restaurant Simple Suppers: Fresh Ideas for the Weeknight Table

Makes about 5 cups.

2 cups chopped onions
2 garlic cloves, minced or pressed
3 cups diced red potatoes
1 sprig of fresh rosemary (about 4 inches long)
3 cups vegetable broth
1 teaspoon salt
1 14-ounce can of small red beans, drained
½ cup white wine or 2 tablespoons lemon juice (I prefer the taste with
        lemon juice.)
4 ounces arugula (I used spinach) (about 4 cups)
¼ cup chopped, fresh basil
salt and black pepper
lemon wedges (optional)

In a soup pot, sauté the onions and garlic in a little bit of water for about 2 minutes. If the onions begin to stick, add a little bit more water. Add the potatoes, rosemary, broth, and salt. Cover and bring to a boil. Add the beans and the wine. Reduce the heat and simmer, covered, until the potatoes are tender, about 10 minutes.

While the potatoes cook, rinse and drain the arugula. Remove any large or tough stems and coarsely chop any large leaves. Set aside.

When the potatoes are tender, add the basil, salt, and pepper to taste. Remove and discard the rosemary sprig-some leaves may stay behind in the soup, and that's fine. Put a handful of arugula into each bowl and ladle the hot soup over it. Serve immediately with lemon wedges.

Cabbage Soup
From my mother, Joan Trombetta

6 large green onions, chopped
2-4 cans whole tomatoes
1 large head of cabbage, shredded
2 green bell peppers, diced
celery, diced
any kind of dried soup mix
2-3 carrots, chopped

Season to taste with salt, pepper, curry powder, parsley, vegetable bouillon, or hot sauce. Add water to cover and boil until tender.

Carrot and Red Pepper Soup
From Physicians Committee for Responsible Medicine's 21-Day Vegan Kick Start Program

Makes 4 1 ½ cup servings.

1 onion, chopped
6 carrots, thinly sliced
2 cups water or vegetable stock
2 red bell peppers
2 cups non-dairy milk
2 teaspoons lemon juice
2 teaspoons balsamic vinegar
½ teaspoon salt
¼ teaspoon freshly ground black pepper

Place onion and carrots into a pot with water or stock and simmer, covered, over medium heat until the carrots can be easily pierced with a fork, about 20 minutes.

Roast bell peppers by placing them over an open gas flame or directly under the broiler until the skin is completely blackened. Place in a bowl, cover, and let stand about 15 minutes. Slip the charred skin off with your fingers, then cut the peppers in half and remove the seeds.

Blend the carrot mixture along with the bell peppers in a blender or food processor in several small batches. Add some of the non-dairy milk to each batch to facilitate blending. Return to the pot and add some lemon juice, vinegar, salt, and black pepper. Heat until steamy.

36 calories/cup

Zuppa Vegana: Italian Potato, Bean, and Kale Soup
From Susan Voisin, FatFree Vegan Kitchen
http://blog.fatfreevegan.com/2014/02/zuppa-vegana-italian-potato-bean-and-kale-soup.html

Susan has asked that her recipes not be re-posted. Please follow the link above for the recipe.

Lifting Lemon-Garlic Rice and Lentil Soup
From Kathy Patalsky
http://kblog.lunchboxbunch.com/2014/04/lifting-lemon-garlic-rice-lentil-soup.html

Serves about 4 generous servings

Lentils:

½ cup dry lentils (LePuy lentils were used, but any lentil or bean can be used.)
2 cups vegetable broth

Rice:

1 cup dry short-grain brown rice
2 cups water
pinch of salt

Soup Base:

4-6 cups vegetable broth (depending upon how brothy you'd like it)
4-5 small or 2-3 medium juice lemons, juiced (about ½ cup lemon juice total)
¼ teaspoon lemon zest
½ - 1 teaspoon turmeric
4-5 cloves garlic, chopped
1 bay leaf
¼ teaspoon black pepper
1-2 teaspoon extra virgin olive oil, optional (I did not use and it tasted fine.)
¼ cup flat-leaf parsley, finely chopped

Optional:

2-8 tablespoons nutritional yeast (to taste)

Garnish:

4-6 thin lemon slices

There are two ways to prepare this soup. The first way would be to pile everything in a large soup pot, bring to a boil, and simmer on low until the lentils and rice are tender and you are ready to serve the soup. The second way is to prepare the lentils and rice separately ahead of time, then add the cooked rice and lentils along with the other ingredients to create a soup. This method is detailed below.

Start off by pre-soaking your lentils for fastest cooking. Soak in warm salted water for about two hours before cooking. If you do not pre-soak you can still slow-simmer the lentils until tender, they will just take longer to cook. If soaked, drain lentils and add to a small soup pot along with two cups of vegetable broth. Bring to a boil and then reduce heat to low and simmer for about 20 minutes or until the lentils are tender. If the lentils are not pre-soaked, the simmering time will be about 30-40 minutes.

Kathy used LePuy French lentils in this soup. She said they stay nice and al dente even after cooking so they are not soggy at all. If you can find these lentils, she suggests giving them a try. If not, any lentils will work fine. Lentils are rich in protein, iron, vitamins, and minerals so embrace them in your meals every chance you get!

Prepare the rice in a separate pot while you are cooking the lentils. Bring 2 cups of water, plus a pinch of salt to a boil, add the brown rice, cover with a lid, and reduce to a simmer. Simmer on low for about 30 minutes or until tender and most of the liquid has been absorbed. For soup, you do not need to worry about making rice fluffy or waiting for all of the liquid to be absorbed, since it will be rehydrated by the soup broth anyway.

When the rice and lentils are cooked, you can add them to a large soup pot along with the remaining soup ingredients: lemon juice and zest, garlic, bay leaf, spices, parsley, and broth. Bring to a low boil, then reduce heat to low and simmer until ready to serve. You can add the nutritional yeast now or just before serving each bowl. Remove the bay leaf before serving. Adjust salt, pepper, turmeric, and cayenne to taste if desired.

Serve warm with lemon slices as a garnish in the soup.

Quick and Easy Potato Soup
From Susan Voisin, FatFree Vegan Kitchen
http://blog.fatfreevegan.com/2009/02/quick-and-easy-potato-soup.html

Susan has asked that her recipes not be re-posted. Please follow the link above for the recipe.

Leek, Spinach, and Potato Soup
From The Cancer Project's Food for Life Weekly Recipe

Makes 4 2-cup servings.

1 pound leeks
1 pound fresh spinach, kale, or Swiss chard
6 cups low-sodium or homemade vegetable broth, divided
2 medium Yukon gold potatoes, peeled and chopped (I don't peel them
      and it turns out just fine.)
freshly ground black pepper, to taste
¼ cup non-dairy milk
1 teaspoon dried tarragon
I add salt to taste as well.

Cut off root ends of leeks and remove 1/3 of the green tops. Cut leeks in half lengthwise and slice very thinly. Place leeks in colander and rinse well under cold water. Thoroughly wash spinach, kale, or Swiss chard and remove stems.

Heat about 2 tablespoons broth in a soup pot over medium heat. Add leeks and cook, stirring until they begin to soften, about 6 to 7 minutes. Add spinach and 2 cups broth. Cook for 1 to 2 minutes. Add potatoes and remaining broth. Season with black pepper and bring to a boil. Reduce heat to low and simmer, uncovered, for 30 to 35 minutes.

Next, puree soup in food processor or use an immersion blender for pureeing. After pureeing, return soup to medium-low simmer, and add non-dairy milk and tarragon, and simmer for a few minutes. Taste, adjust seasonings, and serve. I also add salt to taste.

Note: This soup can be prepared several hours or a couple of days ahead. Cover and refrigerate. Reheat soup gently just before serving.

Per serving: 130 calories; 0.6 g fat; 0.1 g saturated fat; 4.2% calories from fat; 0 mg cholesterol; 4.5 g protein; 28.9 g carbohydrate; 6.9 g sugar; 4.1 g fiber; 502 mg sodium; 147 mg calcium; 3.6 mg iron; 15.6 mg vitamin C; 4975 mcg beta-carotene; 2 mg vitamin E

Mexican Corn Chowder
From Healthy Eating for Life to Prevent and Treat Cancer by Physicians Committee for Responsible Medicine with Vesanto Melina, M.S., R.D.

Makes 10 servings.

2-3 cups peeled and chopped potatoes (I leave the skins on.)
2 cups vegetable broth or water
1 yellow onion, chopped
2 garlic cloves, minced
1 red bell pepper, seeded and chopped
1 teaspoon ground cumin
1 teaspoon dried basil
½ teaspoon salt (I use ¼ teaspoon more.)
¼ teaspoon turmeric
¼ teaspoon black pepper (I use ¼ teaspoon more.)
2 15-ounce cans corn (1 can undrained, 1 can drained)
1 4-ounce can diced green chilies
1-2 cups non-dairy milk

Place potatoes in a pot with broth or water. Cover and simmer until tender, about 20 minutes.

In a separate pan, heat ½ cup water and cook onion, garlic, and bell pepper over medium heat until soft, about 5 minutes. Add cumin, basil, salt, turmeric, and black pepper and cook 5 minutes, stirring often.

When potatoes are tender, mash them in their cooking liquid and add onion mixture.

Blend one can of corn, with its liquid, until smooth, 2-3 minutes, then add it to the soup.

Add remaining can of corn, diced chilies, and 1 cup of non-dairy milk. Stir to mix. Add more non-dairy milk if a thinner soup is desired.

Heat gently until very hot and steamy.

Per serving (1 cup): 112 calories, 1.4 g fat, 0.2 g saturated fat, 10.8% calories from fat, 0 mg cholesterol, 4 g protein, 23.7 g carbohydrates, 4.8 g sugar, 3.2 g fiber, 347 mg sodium, 54 mg calcium, 1.6 mg iron, 32.2 mg vitamin C, 428 mcg beta-carotene, 0.7 mg vitamin E

Speedy International Stew
From The McDougall Quick and Easy Cookbook: Over 300 Delicious Low-Fat Recipes You Can Prepare in Fifteen Minutes or Less by Mary and John McDougall, MD

Preparation Time: 5 minutes
Cooking Time: 5 minutes
Makes 4 servings

Keep the ingredients in your pantry for when you have absolutely no time to make something for lunch or dinner.

2 14.5-ounce cans stewed tomatoes (Italian, Mexican, or Cajun)
1 15-ounce can black beans, drained and rinsed
1 16-ounce can corn kernels, drained and rinsed

Place all ingredients in a medium saucepan and cook over medium heat for 5 minutes, stirring occasionally.

Serve with a loaf of fresh bread and a simple green salad for a hearty, quick meal.

Peruvian Quinoa Stew
From Moosewood Restaurant Cooks at Home

Serves 4

½ cup quinoa (I use the pre-rinsed variety.)
1 cup water
2 cups chopped onions
2 garlic cloves, minced or pressed
2 tablespoons vegetable oil
1 celery stalk, chopped
1 carrot, cut on the diagonal into ¼" thick slices
1 bell pepper, cut into 1" pieces
1 cup cubed zucchini
2 cups undrained chopped fresh or canned tomatoes
1 cup water or vegetable stock
2 teaspoons ground cumin
½ teaspoon chili powder
1 teaspoon ground coriander
pinch of cayenne (or more to taste, I used a lot more)
2 teaspoons fresh oregano (1 teaspoon dried)
salt to taste
chopped fresh cilantro (optional)

Using a fine sieve, rinse the quinoa well. Place in a pot with the water and cook, covered, on medium-low heat for about 15 minutes, until soft. Set aside.

While the quinoa cooks, in a covered soup pot sauté the onions and garlic in the oil for about 5 minutes on medium heat. Add the celery and carrots, and continue to cook for 5 minutes, stirring often. Add the bell pepper, zucchini, tomatoes, and water or stock. Stir in the cumin, chili powder, coriander, cayenne, and oregano (I am very generous with the spices.), and simmer, covered, about 10 to 15 minutes, until the vegetables are tender. Stir the cooked quinoa into the stew and add salt to taste. Top with cilantro, if you wish. Serve immediately.

Per 8-oz. serving: 140 calories, 2.8 g protein, 4.7 g fat, 22.9 g carbohydrate, 52 mg sodium, 0 mg cholesterol

Curried Potato Stew
From Jeff Novick, MS, RD, LD, LN

4 small potatoes, diced
1 ½ pounds frozen, mixed vegetables
1 14-ounce can garbanzo beans
1 28-ounce can chopped tomatoes
curry powder
garlic

Let the potatoes simmer for a few minutes in the tomatoes until soft.

Add all other ingredients and cook five more minutes.

Add spices and enjoy!

Now Jeff appears to be one of those wonderful cooks who doesn't need to measure his spices when cooking. I can't do that. For this recipe, I started out with 2 teaspoons curry powder, ¾ teaspoon garlic powder, and ½ teaspoon salt. However, I added more every time I had some. This dish tastes even better the next day!

Kapusta
From Tracey Eakin

1 bag of split peas
1 large can of sauerkraut
vinegar
pepper
salt

Boil split peas until mushy, about 30-45 minutes, adding water as needed. Meanwhile, simmer sauerkraut and its juice for about 30 minutes until tender. Puree peas in a blender. Add sauerkraut to peas in a pot. Add some vinegar, pepper, salt, if necessary.

If a chunkier soup is desired, do not puree the split peas.

Sandwiches, Burgers, and Quesadillas

3-2-1 Hummus
From Kathy Patalsky

http://kblog.lunchboxbunch.com/2014/04/3-2-1-hummus.html?utm_source=feedburner&utm_medium=email&utm_campaign=Feed%3A+KathysBlogHealthyHappyLife+%28Kathy%27s+Blog%3A+Healthy.+Happy.+Life.%29

Makes about 2 cups.

3 tablespoons tahini
2 cups chickpeas, drained and rinsed in warm water
1 large lemon, juiced
water or more lemon juice, if necessary, to thin the hummus

Optional:

salt and pepper, to taste
minced garlic
smoked paprika

Add the tahini, chickpeas, and lemon juice to a food processor or blender. Add optional salt, pepper, and minced garlic. Process on low until the mixture starts to smooth out. If needed, add a splash or two of water or lemon juice to loosen the blend. You may also need to stop blending and scrape down the sides of the container to make sure everything blends smoothly. Add in any blend-in ingredients if desired. Blend until smooth. Taste test and adjust salt and pepper if desired. Scoop mixture into an oven-safe dish. Sprinkle with smoky paprika. You can serve room temperature, chill in the refrigerator, or heat in the oven until warm. Use as a dip, sandwich spread, or any way that appeals to you.

Eggless Salad Sandwiches
From The Cancer Survivor's Guide by Neal D. Barnard, MD and Jennifer K. Reilly, RD

Serves 6

1 14 ounce container of low-fat, firm tofu
1 green onion, finely chopped
2 tablespoons pickle relish
2 tablespoons low-fat vegan mayonnaise (Follow Your Heart's Vegenaise is delicious and is available at health food stores)
2 teaspoons yellow mustard
1 teaspoon salt
¼ teaspoon ground cumin
¼ teaspoon ground turmeric
¼ teaspoon garlic powder
12 slices whole-grain bread
6 lettuce leaves
6 tomato slices

Mash the tofu with a fork, potato masher, or your fingers, leaving some chunks.

Stir in the green onion, relish, vegan mayonnaise, mustard, salt, cumin, turmeric, and garlic powder. Spread on the bread and garnish with the lettuce and tomato.

Stored in a covered container in the refrigerator, leftover Eggless Salad (without the bread, lettuce, and tomato) will keep for up to three days.

Nutrition information per serving:

calories: 175; fat: 3 g; saturated fat: 0.6 g; calories from fat: 15.6%; cholesterol: 0 mg; protein: 9.1 g; carbohydrate: 30.5 g; sugar: 8.9 g; fiber: 4.4 g; sodium: 827 mg; calcium: 67 mg; iron: 2.6 mg; vitamin C: 3.5 mg; beta-carotene: 127 mcg; vitamin E: 0.4 mg

"Chicken" Salad Sandwich
From Skinny Bitch in the Kitch by Rory Freedman and Kim Barnouin

Makes 3 or 4 sandwiches

½ cup vegan mayonnaise
2 teaspoons lemon juice
1 tablespoon course nutritional yeast
½ tablespoon agave nectar
¼ teaspoon fine sea salt
¼ teaspoon curry powder
1/8 teaspoon pepper
2 cups chopped or shredded vegan chicken strips or chunks (thawed, if
        frozen)(I use 4 Quorn naked cutlets which aren't ENTIRELY
        vegan)
¼ cup halved (quartered if large) seedless red grapes (optional)
1 celery stalk, finely diced
¼ small red or white onion, finely diced
2 tablespoons chopped fresh Italian parsley
6 to 8 slice vegan whole wheat bread

In a small bowl, combine the mayonnaise, lemon juice, yeast, agave nectar, salt, curry powder, and pepper. In a large bowl, combine the chicken, grapes (if using), celery, onion, and parsley. Add the mayonnaise mixture to the chicken mixture, tossing gently.

Spread the chicken salad on 3 or 4 slices of bread, top with remaining 3 or 4 slices, and serve.

Can also be served on a bed of lettuce.

660 calories for entire chicken salad recipe, not including bread.

Savory Sandwiches
From John McDougall, MD

Serves: 4
Preparation Time: 15 minutes
Chilling Time: 1 hour

1 15-ounce can garbanzo beans, drained and rinsed
½ cup finely chopped celery
¼ cup finely chopped sweet onion
¼ cup finely chopped green onions
2 tablespoons sweet or dill pickle relish
1 tablespoon lemon juice
¼ cup low-fat vegan mayonnaise (Follow Your Heart's Vegenaise is
      delicious and available at health food stores)
8 slices whole wheat bread
lettuce
tomatoes
mustard

Mash beans with a bean masher. Place in a bowl and add celery, onions, relish, lemon juice, and vegan mayonnaise. Mix well. Chill to blend flavors.

Spread bread with mustard, if desired. Place about ½ cup of the spread on four of the bread slices. Add lettuce, tomatoes, and other slices of bread.

Mock Tuna Salad
From Uma Purighalla, MD

1 can garbanzo beans, drained and rinsed
2 tablespoons relish
1 celery stalk, chopped
2 tablespoons Follow Your Heart's Original Vegenaise (available in
      health food stores and most grocery stores)
1/8 teaspoon salt

Mash or blend the garbanzo beans, then mix in remaining ingredients. Serve on flourless Ezekiel bread or whole wheat tortillas and add baby arugula and chopped tomatoes.

Colleen's Chickpea Burgers with Tahini Sauce
From Susan Voisin, FatFree Vegan Kitchen
http://blog.fatfreevegan.com/2011/10/colleens-chickpea-
burgers-with-tahini-sauce.html

Susan has asked that her recipes not be re-posted. Please follow the
link above for the recipe.

BBQ Peanut Sweet Potato Burgers
From Kathy Patalsky
http://kblog.lunchboxbunch.com/2013/03/spin-on-sweet-potato-veggie-burgers-bbq.html?utm_source=feedburner&utm_medium=email&utm_campaign=Feed%3A+KathysBlogHealthyHappyLife+%28Kathy%27s+Blog%3A+Healthy.+Happy.+Life.%29

These patties are very tasty but they don't hold together as well as I would like. They do tend to fuse and firm up a little as they cool. The next night, I served it heated like mashed potatoes instead of forming patties and baking them and it was unique but tasty.

Makes 5-6 patties

½ cup cooked brown rice, short grain (I don't know if I used short or long grain but it seemed to work nonetheless)
½ - ¾ cup whole peanuts, roasted and salted (process into crumbly bits), start with ½ cup and add more if you like a nuttier burger
1 cup mashed sweet potato
1 ½ cups cannellini white beans, drained and rinsed in hot water to soften
1 tablespoon dry BBQ spice blend
2 tablespoons liquid vegan BBQ sauce
¼ cup onion, diced
2 tablespoons flat leaf parsley, finely chopped
¼ teaspoon fine black pepper
½ teaspoon garlic powder
a few dashes cayenne (optional)
salt to taste

oil for baking or sautéing
vegan burger buns
vegan mayo (Follow Your Heart's Original Vegenaise is available at health food stores and most grocery stores)
sliced avocado (tossed in lemon juice to prevent browning)
vegan cole slaw (optional topping or possible side dish)
sliced onions
sliced tomatoes

mixed greens
warmed BBQ sauce
regular or sweet potato tater tots

Preheat oven to 400 degrees F.

Prep your veggies, process your peanuts, and cook your rice. I used my Vitamix to process my peanuts. You'll want a blend of fine crumbles that range from powdery to chunky.

Combine the sweet potato, rice, beans, peanuts, spices, onion, parsley, and BBQ sauce in a large mixing bowl. Mash until the mixture is thick and creamy.

Place a small amount of oil on a paper towel and spread sparingly on a baking sheet. This is a must to prevent sticking. Bake at 400 degrees F for about 15 minutes or until the edges brown. If you like your patties on the softer side, just undercook them a bit. If sautéing, add a splash of oil to a hot sauté pan and cook 2-4 minutes on each side over medium-high heat. Patties will fuse and firm up as they cool.

Try toasting your buns, slathering warmed BBQ sauce on one side and vegan mayo on the other. Place the patty, onions, sliced tomatoes, sliced avocados, and greens on top, slice, and enjoy. Try serving with a side of vegan cole slaw and regular or sweet potato tater tots.

Sloppy Joes
From Ecological Cooking: Recipes to Save the Planet

Serves 4 for a meal, with leftovers for another.

2 large green bell peppers, diced
1 large yellow onion, chopped
2-3 cloves garlic, minced
3 tablespoons olive oil (reduce as your tastes adapt to lower fat cook
      ing)
2 cups textured vegetable protein (TVP) rehydrated in 1 ¾ cup boiling
      water
1 16-ounce can tomato puree
1 cup tomatoes, diced
¼ teaspoon basil
¼ teaspoon oregano
¼ teaspoon paprika
¼ teaspoon salt
freshly ground black pepper
2 tablespoons Worcestershire sauce

I like this recipe even spicier so I doubled all of the spices, then added cayenne pepper, ketchup, hot taco sauce, garlic salt, and extra paprika.

In a large saucepan, sauté peppers, onions, and garlic in oil until soft. Add TVP and brown lightly, stirring often and adding water, if needed, to keep from sticking. Add remaining ingredients and simmer about an hour until flavors are absorbed. Serve in buns.

Note: For a faster meal, combine one 12-ounce bag of Beyond Meat frozen meatless ground crumbles with one can of sloppy Joe sauce and heat in either the microwave or on the stove top. Always try to add extra vegetables into your meal. Try chopping a small onion and a large green pepper into the meatless crumbles. It adds taste and additional vegetables too!

Homemade Pizza

There are a number of homemade whole wheat pizza dough recipes on the Internet, but a whole wheat Boboli pizza crust works too. Slather on your favorite pizza sauce and load it up with your favorite vegetables.

If you miss the cheese, you can sprinkle a little Daiya cheese shreds on top of the sauce before you add your vegetables.

Pizza doesn't have to be off limits. Enjoy!

Casseroles

No Fuss Casserole
From Tracey Eakin

3 cups instant brown rice, cooked according to directions
3 cups of frozen corn, cooked
1 15-ounce can of kidney beans, or any other bean that you like, rinsed
   and drained
1 6-ounce can of small, pitted, whole black olives, drained
2 16-ounce jars of your favorite salsa
low-fat guacamole (I love Giant Eagle's spicy guacamole.)

Cook the rice and corn and combine with the beans, black olives, and salsa in a large casserole dish. Serve topped with guacamole and enjoy! Can be coupled with a salad, steamed vegetables, and applesauce.

Potato and Veggie Casserole
From Keep it Simple, Keep it Whole: Your Guide to Optimum Health by Alona Pulde, MD and Matthew Lederman, MD

4 cups vegan broth
1-2 garlic cloves
2 carrots, chopped
1 celery stalk, chopped
1 small onion, diced
1 cup green beans
1 ½ cups mushrooms (I prefer portabellas for a heartier taste), sliced
1 ½ cups corn, fresh or frozen
½ teaspoon marjoram
¼ teaspoon sage
2 teaspoons Bragg's Liquid Aminos
2 tablespoons cornstarch mixed with 1/3 cup cold water
4 large Yukon gold potatoes, peeled (3-4 cups mashed)
salt and pepper to taste
¼ cup nutritional yeast, if desired (I always add.)

1. Place potatoes in a pot and boil until tender. Drain the potatoes and place in a bowl for later.
2. In a small amount of broth, sauté garlic, carrots, celery, and onion until softened.
3. Add remaining vegetables, spices, and broth and simmer until soft.
4. Blend the cornstarch or potato starch mixed with water and bring vegetables to a boil, stirring until thickened. Place in a casserole dish.
5. Mash the potatoes adding water or vegetable broth as needed to achieve desired consistency.
6. Season with salt and pepper.
7. Stir in ¼ cup nutritional yeast, if desired for a richer taste.
8. Spread potatoes on top of vegetables.
9. Sprinkle with paprika and bake at 350 for 30 minutes or until bubbling. You can briefly broil the top to crisp the potatoes.

Note: This is an extremely versatile recipe. You can use any combination of vegetables. The addition of extra mushrooms seems to please the meat eater who is adjusting his/her palate.

Red Bean Casserole
From The Cancer Survivor's Guide by Neal D. Barnard, MD and Jennifer K. Reilly, RD

This is a very simple dish. It doesn't contain a sauce or a lot of spices. I think it is for this reason that it is such a hit with children.

Serves 4

3 cups cooked long-grain brown rice
3 cups cooked or canned red beans, rinsed and drained
1 cup diced red onion
1 cup diced celery
2 tablespoons minced fresh parsley
1 teaspoon salt
1 garlic clove, minced or pressed
½ teaspoon ground black pepper
Dash of hot sauce

Preheat the oven to 350 degrees F.

Combine all of the ingredients in a 9x13-inch casserole dish and mix until evenly combined. Bake uncovered for 20 minutes, or until heated through.

Stored in a covered container in the refrigerator, leftover Red Bean Casserole will keep for up to 3 days.

Per serving: 344 calories; 1.2 g fat; 0.3 g saturated fat; 3.2% calories from fat; 0 mg cholesterol; 15.2 g protein; 68.5 g total carbohydrate; 2.9 g sugar; 8 g fiber; 967 mg sodium; 71 mg calcium; 5.5 mg iron; 6.9 mg vitamin C; 204 mcg beta-carotene; 0.6 mg vitamin E

Asparagus and Chickpea Casserole
From Susan Voisin, FatFree Vegan Kitchen
http://blog.fatfreevegan.com/2010/09/asparagus-and-chickpea-casserole.html

Children love this recipe!

Susan has asked that her recipes not be re-posted. Please follow the link above for the recipe.

Creamy Vegan Broccoli and Rice Casserole
From Susan Voisin, FatFree Vegan Kitchen
http://blog.fatfreevegan.com/2011/11/creamy-vegan-broccoli-and-rice-casserole.html

Susan has asked that her recipes not be re-posted. Please follow the link above for the recipe.

Cheezy Casserole
From Skinny Bitch in the Kitch by Rory Freedman and Kim Barnouin

Serves 6-8.

Refined coconut oil, for the casserole dish
1 ½ cups short grain brown rice
3 quarts plus 3 cups water
About 4 ¾ teaspoons fine sea salt
8 ounces (or four to six) red potatoes, cut into ¾-inch cubes
2 carrots, cut on a diagonal into ¼-inch slices
½ red onion, cut into ¾-inch dice
4 ounces sugar snap peas, cut crosswise in half
1 broccoli crown, cut into bite-sized florets (about 2 ½ cups)
14 to 16 ounces firm, extra firm, or baked tofu, cut into ½-inch cubes
2 ¾ cups Cheezy Sauce (recipe found later in this book)
¼ cup coarsely chopped Italian parsley
1/3 cup sliced almonds
Tamari or soy sauce, for serving (optional)

Preheat oven to 375 degrees F. Grease a 2-quart casserole dish. Line a large bowl with one or two paper towels.

In a 2-quart saucepan over high heat, combine rice, 3 cups of the water, and ¼ teaspoon of the salt. Bring to a boil, reduce the heat to a simmer, cover, and cook until the water is absorbed and the rice is tender, about 45 minutes. Remove from heat and let the rice stand, covered, at least 10 minutes.

Meanwhile, in a 4- to 6-quart stockpot over high heat, combine the remaining 3 quarts of water with about 1 ½ tablespoons salt. Bring the water to a boil. Add the potatoes and cook until they care soft but still holding their shape, about 5 minutes. Use a slotted spoon or hand-held strainer to remove the potatoes to the prepared bowl. Then remove the paper towels. Add the carrots and onion to the stockpot and cook until tender, about 2 minutes. Use the same slotted spoon to remove the carrots and onions, adding them to the bowl. Add the snap peas and broccoli to the stockpot and cook until tender, about 1 minute. Remove the snap peas and broccoli, adding them to the bowl.

Add the rice, tofu, Cheezy Sauce, and parsley to the vegetables, tossing until combined. Transfer the mixture to the prepared casserole dish. Place the casserole on a rimmed baking sheet and bake for 30 minutes. Sprinkle almonds on top and bake for 15 minutes, or until the almonds are toasted and the tip of a knife inserted into the center of the casserole comes out piping hot. If using, pass the tamari or soy sauce at the table.

Other Entrees and Side Dishes

Southern Stir-Fry
From Betty Crocker Easy Vegetarian
www.youtube.com/watch?v=e2_Ko6QKCM0

Preparation Time: 7 minutes
Cook Time: 6 minutes
Makes 4 servings.

1 tablespoon vegetable oil (this can be weaned down to ½ tablespoon)
1 cup cold cooked brown rice
1 cup frozen whole kernel corn
1 ½ teaspoons chopped fresh or ½ teaspoon dried thyme leaves
½ teaspoon garlic salt
1/8 teaspoon cayenne pepper
1 15-16 ounce can black-eyed peas, rinsed and drained
2 cups lightly packed spinach leaves (you can use A LOT more)

Heat wok or 12-inch skillet over medium-high heat. Add oil; rotate to coat sides.

Add all ingredients except spinach to skillet; stir-fry 3-4 minutes or until heated through. Add spinach; stir-fry 1-2 minutes or until spinach begins to wilt.

Per Serving:

205 calories
25 calories from fat
3 g fat (1 g saturated fat)
0 mg cholesterol
350 mg sodium
42 g carbohydrate
8g dietary fiber
11 g protein

Parsnip Mashed Potatoes
From The Cancer Survivor's Guide by Neal D. Barnard, MD and Jennifer K. Reilly, RD

Makes 4 1-cup servings.

3 whole garlic cloves, peeled
1 parsnip, peeled and cut into 1" chunks
2 large russet potatoes, cut into 1" chunks
¾ cup water
½ cup plain, unsweetened non-dairy milk
½ teaspoon salt
1/8 teaspoon ground black pepper

Place the garlic in a medium saucepan. Arrange the parsnip over the garlic. Then arrange the potatoes over the parsnip. Add the water and bring to a simmer over medium heat. Reduce the heat to low, cover, and cook for about 25 minutes, until the parsnips and potatoes are tender when pierced with a knife. Check occasionally and add more water, 1 tablespoon at a time, if the saucepan becomes too dry.

Mash with a potato masher, a fork, or automatic blender. Then stir in enough non-dairy milk to obtain a creamy consistency. Season with salt and pepper to taste.

Stored in a covered container in the refrigerator, leftover Parsnip Mashed Potatoes will keep for up to 2 days.

Per 1 cup serving: 161 calories; 0.6 g fat; 0.1 g saturated fat; 3.4% calories from fat; 0 mg cholesterol; 4.1 g protein; 36.1 g carbohydrates; 3 g sugar; 4.3 g fiber; 328 mg sodium; 63 mg calcium; 0.9 mg iron; 15.1 mg vitamin C; 3 mcg beta-carotene; 0.3 mg vitamin E

Mashed NOtatoes
From Unprocessed by Chef AJ

1 head of cauliflower
nutritional yeast, to taste

Steam or blanch cauliflower until soft. Place cauliflower in a food processor fitted with the "S" blade and process until smooth and creamy. Add seasonings to taste and process again (I add pepper as well.).

This is a great recipe for many reasons. It is not supposed to replace mashed potatoes because potatoes are one of the healthiest foods you can eat. It is simply a great alternative way to serve cauliflower. Cauliflower may be more appealing to children when presented this way. In addition, if you have cancer and are trying to increase your intake of cruciferous vegetables, eating a large serving of cauliflower in this form is much easier to me than sitting down to a huge plate of steamed cauliflower. It also provides the sensation that you're eating a comfort food. It's creamy and savory and very satisfying. Chef AJ swears with a little gravy on top that no one will know they're not mashed potatoes. I don't know that I would agree, but this recipe is delicious for whatever reason you are making it.

Tex Mex Potatoes with Tofu Taco Topping
From The Starch Solution

Serves 6

Tex Mex Potatoes:

6 large red potatoes, cut lengthwise into wedges
2 15-ounce cans pinto beans, drained and rinsed
1 cup salsa
1 4-ounce can chopped green chilies
1 small onion, chopped
1-2 cloves garlic, crushed or minced
½ teaspoon chili powder
½ teaspoon ground cumin
¼ cup chopped fresh cilantro, divided
1 tomato, chopped
¼ cup fresh or frozen and thawed corn kernels
2 scallions (green and white parts), chopped

Preheat oven to 375 degrees F. Place the potatoes on a baking sheet and bake until lightly browned, about 40 minutes.

While the potatoes cook, in a saucepan, stir together the beans, salsa, chilies, onion, garlic, chili powder, cumin, and half of the cilantro. Cook over low heat, stirring occasionally, for 15 minutes.

Stir together the tomato, corn, scallions, and the remaining cilantro in a small bowl.

To serve, arrange the baked potato wedges on a serving platter. Spoon the warm bean mixture over them and top with the fresh tomato mixture. Garnish with several dollops of Tofu Taco Topping (recipe follows), if desired.

Tofu Taco Topping:

This topping also makes a very good dip for cooked, chilled potato chunks or raw vegetables.

1 12.3-ounce package silken tofu, drained in a fine mesh strainer
½ - 1 packet taco seasoning mix

Combine the tofu and seasoning mix in a food processor until very smooth. Taste, and add more of the taco seasoning for a spicier flavor, if desired. Transfer to a bowl.

For best flavor, cover and chill for several hours before serving.

Sweet Potato and Blue Corn Enchiladas
From Unprocessed by Chef AJ

Sauce Ingredients:

1 red onion, chopped
2 cloves garlic, crushed
1 28-ounce can salt-free tomatoes
3 tablespoons chili powder
1 teaspoon cumin
3 tablespoons arrowroot powder
1 tablespoon low sodium tamari (I use Bragg Liquid Aminos.)
1 ½ cups water

Preheat oven to 350 degrees F.

Place the onion, garlic, and liquid in a pot and cook 8-10 minutes until soft. Stir in tomato and spices and cook on low heat for 15 minutes. Add tamari and arrowroot powder and stir until thickened.

Filling Ingredients:

2 cups Pico de Gallo or store-bought, salt-free salsa
3 cups sweet potatoes
1 pound bag frozen roasted corn, defrosted (I use regular frozen corn.)
12 blue corn tortillas (I use sprouted ancient grain tortillas.) (I only use
      7 tortillas.)
Topping: sliced olives and scallions (optional)

Peel sweet potatoes and boil, steam, or microwave until soft. Mash. Stir in remainder of ingredients.

Cover the bottom of the baking dish with half of the enchilada sauce. Spread sweet potato filling down the center of each tortilla. Roll up and place seam side down in the dish. Pour the remaining sauce over the tortillas and sprinkle with sliced olives, if using, over the top. Bake for 30 minutes. Sprinkle with scallions and top with guacamole, if desired.

Italian Mushrooms
Adapted from my mother, Joan Trombetta

white mushrooms
1-2 cups water or enough so that it doesn't boil down
salt (be generous, but not too much)
pepper
oregano (the primary spice)
garlic salt
a little Italian Seasoning

Bring to a boil and simmer until the mushrooms are gray and tender.

Spaghetti with Zucchini and Lemon
From Moosewood Restaurant Cooks at Home

Preparation and Cook Time: 25 minutes
Makes 4-6 servings.

1 pound spaghetti or linguine
1 tablespoon olive oil
4 garlic cloves, minced or pressed
6-8 small, tender, young zucchini, sliced (4 cups or you can use more)
dash of salt and ground black pepper
juice of 1 lemon
6 large, fresh basil leaves, cut into thin strips

Bring a large, covered pot of water to a rapid boil. Add the pasta, stir briefly, and cover the pot until the water boils again. Uncover the pot.

While the pasta cooks, heat the olive oil in a large, heavy, nonreactive skillet. Add the garlic and zucchini, and sauté on medium-high heat until the zucchini begins to brown. Sprinkle with salt and pepper. Add the lemon juice and basil, stir, and remove from the heat. The zucchini should be done just before the pasta is ready. When the pasta is al dente, drain it and place it in a large, warmed serving bowl. Toss it with zucchini and serve immediately.

Raw Vegan Pesto with Zucchini Noodles
From Tracy Russell at
http://www.incrediblesmoothies.com/raw-food-diet/raw-recipes/raw-vegan-pesto-with-zucchini-noodles/

Serves 1

½ cup tomatoes, soaked for about 20 minutes (I didn't soak them and
     they were okay.)
½ to 1 clove minced garlic
½ teaspoon nutritional yeast
Juice from 1 small lime
Dash of sea salt (or to taste)
¼ cup fresh basil
¼ cup raw pine nuts
4 pieces of sun-dried tomatoes
1 medium zucchini

Add the tomatoes, garlic, nutritional yeast, lime juice, sea salt, basil, and pine nuts to your blender or food processor and blend until creamy. Once finished, set aside while you wash the zucchini and remove the ends.

Using a spiral slicer, turn the zucchini into "noodles". If you do not have a spiral slicer, you can use a julienne or mandolin slicer (with a julienne blade). If you don't have any spiral slicers, you can use a simple cheese grater. Simply shred the zucchini lengthwise into long, flat noodles.

This is the spiralizer I have and I love it:

http://www.amazon.com/gp/product/B0007Y9WHQ/ref=oh_details_o03_s00_i00?ie=UTF8&psc=1

Once the zucchini is turned into noodles, toss with the pesto sauce and top with chopped sun-dried tomatoes, mushrooms, or the topping of your choice.

Zucchini "Noodles" with Sesame-Peanut Sauce
From Susan Voisin, FatFree Vegan Kitchen
http://blog.fatfreevegan.com/2013/04/zucchini-noodles-with-sesame-peanut-sauce.html

Susan has asked that her recipes not be re-posted. Please follow the link above for the recipe.

This is the spiralizer I have and I love it:

http://www.amazon.com/gp/product/B0007Y9WHQ/ref=oh_details_o03_s00_i00?ie=UTF8&psc=1

Halusky
From Tracey Eakin

1 package of eggless noodles (often called pasta ribbons)
about ½ tablespoon vegetable oil
minced garlic
onion, chopped
cabbage, chopped or shredded
pepper
salt

Prepare noodles. Sauté minced garlic, onion, and sliced cabbage in oil until tender. Season with pepper and salt to taste. Toss noodles with cabbage mix and season with pepper and salt to taste.

Easy Thai Noodles
From Chef Del Sroufe

Makes about 7 cups.
Ready in 30 minutes.

8 ounces brown rice noodles or other whole grain noodles
3 tablespoons low-sodium soy sauce, or to taste
2 tablespoons brown rice syrup or agave nectar (I prefer to use half this
    amount.)
2 tablespoons fresh lime juice (from 1 to 2 limes)
4 cloves garlic, minced
1 12-ounce package frozen Asian-style vegetables (about 3 cups)
1 cup mung bean sprouts
2 green onions, white and light green parts, chopped
3 tablespoons chopped, roasted, unsalted peanuts
¼ cup chopped fresh cilantro
1 lime, cut into wedges

Cook the noodles according to the package instructions. Drain and set aside.

Meanwhile in a large saucepan, combine the soy sauce, brown rice syrup, lime juice, garlic, and ¼ cup water. Bring to a boil over medium heat. Stir in the Asian mixed vegetables and cook until crisp-tender, about five minutes.

Add the cooked noodles and mung bean sprouts and toss to coat. Cook until heated through, about two minutes.

Garnish the noodles with the green onions, chopped peanuts, cilantro, and lime wedges. Serve.

Hurry-Up Hoisin Tofu and Vegetables with Rice Noodles
From Susan Voisin, FatFree Vegan Kitchen
http://blog.fatfreevegan.com/2006/03/hurry-up-hoisin-tofu-and-vegetables.html

Susan has asked that her recipes not be re-posted. Please follow the link above for the recipe.

Sichuan Tofu with Garlic Sauce
From Susan Voisin, FatFree Vegan Kitchen,
http://blog.fatfreevegan.com/2007/11/sichuan-tofu-with-garlic-sauce.html

Susan has asked that her recipes not be re-posted. Please follow the link above for the recipe.

The garlic sauce in this recipe can be made by itself and used in other Asian meals. It is delicious!

Black Beans and Rice Extravaganza!
From Engine 2 Diet

2 cans black beans, drained and rinsed
1 cup water or vegetable stock
1 tablespoon Bragg Liquid Aminos
1 teaspoon red chili powder
2 to 3 tomatoes, chopped
1 bunch green onions, chopped
1 can water chestnuts, drained
1 cup corn, fresh, frozen, or canned and drained
2 red, yellow, or green bell peppers, seeded and chopped
1 bunch cilantro, rinsed and chopped
1 avocado, peeled and sliced
3 cups cooked brown rice
salsa or tamari, to taste

Heat the beans with the water or broth, Bragg's, and chili powder. Chop vegetables and place in individual bowls. To serve, place several big spoonfuls of brown rice onto large plates and ladle beans on top. Add generous handfuls of chopped vegetables on top of the beans. Sprinkle with cilantro. Add salsa or tamari to taste. Top with avocado slices.

Rice Medley
From The McDougall Quick and Easy Cookbook: Over 300 Delicious Low-Fat Recipes You Can Prepare in Fifteen Minutes or Less by Mary and John McDougall, MD

Makes 6 to 8 servings

½ cup vegetable broth
1 onion, chopped
1 green bell pepper, chopped
½ pound sliced fresh mushrooms
1 bunch green onions, chopped
½ teaspoon minced fresh garlic
1 14.5-ounce can stewed tomatoes
1 4-ounce can chopped green chilies
1 tablespoon soy sauce
1 teaspoon chili powder (I prefer more.)
dash or two of Tabasco sauce (I prefer more.)
4 cups cooked brown rice
¼ cup chopped cilantro

Place the vegetable broth in a large pot. Add the onion, bell pepper, mushrooms, green onions, and garlic. Cook, stirring occasionally, for 5 minutes. Add the remaining ingredients, except the rice and cilantro. Cook, stirring occasionally, for 5 more minutes. Add the rice and cilantro. Cook for an additional 5 minutes. Serve at once.

Recipe Hint: Use one of the seasoned stewed tomatoes, such as Mexican-style, Cajun-style, or Italian-style, for even more flavor in this dish.

North African Couscous Paella
From Moosewood Restaurant Cooks at Home

Total Time: 20 minutes
Serves: 2

½ tablespoon vegetable oil
½ cup chopped red bell pepper
4 scallions, chopped (about ½ cup)
2 garlic cloves, minced or pressed
1 teaspoon ground coriander
½ teaspoon turmeric
pinch of cayenne (I prefer to use more.)

2 cups hot vegetable stock or hot water
¾ pound five-spice tofu, cut into ½-inch cubes
1 cup fresh or frozen green peas
1 cup quick-cooking couscous
½ tablespoon Earth Balance organic buttery spread (available in gro
        cery stores)
salt and ground pepper to taste

coarsely chopped toasted almonds
chopped fresh parsley
lemon wedges

Heat the oil in a 2-quart saucepan. Add the peppers, scallions, garlic,
coriander, turmeric, and cayenne, and sauté on medium heat for 3-4
minutes, stirring occasionally. Stir in the stock or water. Add the tofu
and cook for another 3-4 minutes, until the tofu is hot. Stir in the peas
and cook for another minute. Mix in the couscous and the buttery
spread. Cover, remove from heat, and let stand for 5 minutes.

Uncover the pan and using a fork, stir thoroughly to fluff up the
couscous and break up any lumps. Add salt and pepper to taste. Serve
on a platter, topped with toasted almonds, parsley, and lemon wedges.

For help toasting nuts, please refer to the Helpful Hints chapter.

Sweet Roasted Corn Risotto
From Kathy Patalsky
http://kblog.lunchboxbunch.com/2013/07/sweet-roasted-corn-risotto-cheezy-easy.html

Children love this recipe!

Serves2-3.

Risotto:

1 cup Arborio rice
4-5 cups vegetable broth (or water and additional salt)
pinch of salt
¼ - ½ cup nutritional yeast
dash of black pepper

Corn:

1 ear of corn, kernels sliced off
1 tablespoon sunflower oil
generous seasoning, Kathy uses chili salt and some pepper

Garnish:

chopped parsley and cayenne with black pepper

Accent:

Tofurky Vegan "Beer Brats" sliced and baked in oven alongside corn (optional)

Preheat oven to 400 degrees F.

Slice the kernels off the corn and toss them in the sunflower oil. Add the kernels to a greased baking sheet. Sprinkle the seasoning on top of the kernels.

Place the corn in the oven and bake for about 10 minutes. Then turn oven to broil and broil for another 2-3 minutes, watching closely so the kernels do not burn or start popping! When the kernels start to blacken around a few edges, turn heat off and let them sit in the hot oven while you prepare your risotto. If adding Beer Brats, you can slice and bake in the oven alongside the corn.

Add the rice and 3 cups of vegetable broth and bring to a boil in a large sauté pan or medium soup pot. Once boiling, stir a lot for a minute and then reduce heat to medium and continue to simmering/low boil.

Using a wooden spoon, stir continuously during most of the risotto process. You will spend a good 10 minutes hovering over your rice, but enjoy that meditation time as you prepare your meal. After the liquid is absorbed, you can add more broth (or water) in 1/3 cup portions. Keep adding liquid and stirring. The rice will get soft and velvety. At some point toward the end, add the spices and nutritional yeast. Do a taste test and keep adding liquid if you want the rice to be softer. Stop when you like the texture. You may add more or less liquid to the rice depending on your tastes.

When the rice is ready, you can fold in a small scoop of corn.

To plate, add the risotto to a shallow bowl and top with plenty of roasted corn. Add some parsley and cayenne as desired. Add optional vegan "Beer Brat" slices to plate as desired.

Notes: You could add ½ cup chopped onion or other vegetables to the rice as it is cooking. For a silkier texture, you could add in 1 cup of plain/unsweetened non-dairy milk in place of the vegetable broth during the simmering of the rice. You could also serve the risotto with a splash of soy creamer or non-dairy milk over the top of it.

Rainbow Risotto
From John McDougall, MD

Serves 6

4 cups vegetable broth
1 cup uncooked Arborio rice
1 onion, finely chopped
2 cups broccoli florets
1 cup finely chopped zucchini
1 cup frozen corn kernels, thawed
1 cup finely chopped red bell pepper
1 cup finely chopped green bell pepper
1 tablespoon soy sauce
2 cups chopped spinach
fresh ground pepper to taste

Place 3 ½ cups of broth in a saucepan and bring to a boil. Stir in the rice, reduce heat and cook over low heat, stirring frequently, until broth is absorbed, about 15 minutes.

Meanwhile, place remaining ½ cup of broth in a large non-stick frying pan. Add onions, broccoli, zucchini, corn, and bell pepper. Cook, stirring occasionally for 10 minutes. Add soy sauce and spinach. Cook about 3 minutes. Combine the rice and vegetable mixture. Season with fresh ground pepper.

Easy Vegan Greens and Beans
By Sassy Knutson, Vegan Coach

Serves 2.

1 cup pre-cooked black beans (I use cannellini beans.)
½ cup pre-cooked brown rice (Can omit and it tastes just fine.)
2 tablespoons tamari (I use Bragg Liquid Aminos.)
3-4 cups coarsely chopped Swiss Chard
1-2 tablespoons tomato sauce
dash of red chili powder
1-2 tablespoons Sassy's Seedalicious Topping (recipe below) (I didn't
        use and it tasted fine.)
2 tablespoons nutritional yeast
salt, to taste

In a large, non-stick frying pan with a lid, place the pre-cooked beans and pre-cooked rice, along with about ¼-1/3 cup of bean cooking liquid (or just use water or vegetable broth) and the tamari. Heat over medium heat, stirring occasionally, until warmed. Turn heat down to medium-low, top with Swiss chard, and cover until chard wilts. The liquids you've previously added will help to steam the greens and prevent the grains from sticking.

Add the remaining ingredients and heat, stirring occasionally, until warmed throughout. Serve.

I also cooked garlic and asparagus in the pan and it went with it really well.

Sassy's Seedalicious Topping
From Sassy Knutson, Vegan Coach

Mix 2 parts flax seeds with 1 part each of sunflower, sesame, and pumpkin seeds. Grind 1-2 tablespoons at a time in a coffee grinder or a strong blender like a Vitamix, with a little salt. Can also mix in double the amount of nutritional yeast to the mixture.

Super Vegetarian Chili
From A Physician's Slimming Guide by Neal D. Barnard, MD

Combine in a large saucepan or Dutch oven:

1 28-ounce can crushed whole tomatoes
6 ounce can tomato paste
1 large onion, chopped
1 green pepper, chopped
1 cup textured vegetable protein (TVP), rehydrated with 1 cup boiling
      water or Beyond Meat crumbles can be used instead
1 jalapeno pepper, minced
2 tablespoons (or more) chili powder
1-2 teaspoons (or more) cumin
1 teaspoon garlic powder
1 teaspoon oregano
¼ teaspoon (or more) allspice
salt to taste

Cover pan and simmer for an hour. Taste and add salt if needed. Add:

1 cup red kidney beans

Simmer 30-60 minutes more. Serve on top of mashed potatoes, brown rice, or for an interesting switch, on top of spaghetti. This is even better reheated the next day.

128 calories per cup

Hearty Chili Mac
From Healthy Eating for Life for Children by Amy Lanou, PhD; recipe by Jennifer Raymond, M.S., R.D.

Makes 10 1-cup servings.

8 ounces dry macaroni noodles
½ cup water
1 onion, chopped
3 garlic cloves, minced
1 small red or green pepper, seeded and diced
1 8-ounce package vegan ground beef substitute, or 4 vegan burgers, thawed and chopped
1 28-ounce can crushed tomatoes
1 15-ounce can kidney beans, undrained
1 15-ounce can corn, undrained
2 tablespoons chili powder
1 teaspoon ground cumin
salt
pepper

Cook macaroni according to package directions. Drain, rinse, and set aside.

Heat water in a large pot. Add onion and garlic. Cook until onion is soft, about 5 minutes.

Add bell pepper and vegan ground beef substitute or chopped vegan burgers. Mix in tomatoes, beans and their liquid, corn and its liquid, chili powder, and cumin. Cover and simmer over medium heat, stirring occasionally, for 20 minutes.

Add cooked pasta and check seasonings. Add more chili powder if a spicier dish is desired. Add salt and pepper to taste.

Per 1-cup serving:

211 calories
2.1 g fat

0.3 g saturated fat
8.7% calories from fat
0 mg cholesterol
12 g protein
38.3 g carbohydrates
4.7 g sugar
5.1 g fiber
348 mg sodium
62 mg calcium
3.5 mg iron
23.9 mg vitamin C
450 mcg beta-carotene
1.3 mg vitamin E

Greek-Style Cannellini and Vegetables
From Moosewood Restaurant Cooks at Home

Preparation and Cook Time: 40 minutes
Makes 4 servings.

2 quarts water
2 garlic cloves, minced or pressed
1 large onion, chopped (or about 1 ½ cups)
½ tablespoon olive oil
2-3 carrots (about 2 cups diced)
1 red or green bell pepper
1 cup orzo
1 zucchini (6 inches long)
1 tablespoon minced fresh mint (1 teaspoon dried, I used 2 teaspoons)
1 tablespoon minced fresh dill (1 teaspoon dried, I used 1 ½ table spoons)
½ teaspoon fresh marjoram (sprinkling of dried, I used 1 teaspoon)
5 artichoke hearts, drained and chopped (1 14-ounce can)
1 ½ - 2 cups drained, cooked cannellini or white kidney beans (1 15-ounce can)
1 ½ - 2 cups Italian-style stewed tomatoes (1 14.5-ounce can)
salt and ground black pepper to taste
red wine vinegar

Bring the water to a boil in a large covered pot.

While the water heats, sauté the garlic and onions in the oil in a large skillet on medium-high heat. While the garlic and onions sauté, dice the carrots and chop the pepper. Add them to the onions and stir. When the water boils, add the orzo, return to a boil, and simmer for about 10 minutes, until al dente. Dice the zucchini and stir it into the skillet of vegetables. Add the mint, dill, and marjoram. Add the artichoke hearts. Gently stir in the beans and the stewed tomatoes. Simmer for several minutes, stirring occasionally.

When the pasta is al dente, drain it. When the beans and vegetables are hot, add the orzo. Season with salt and pepper to taste. Serve with a cruet of red wine vinegar at the table for a splash of flavor.

106 calories per 8-oz. serving

Beans Florentine
From The McDougall Quick and Easy Cookbook

Serves 6
Preparation Time: 10 minutes
Cooking Time: 28 minutes

1 onion, chopped
1 stalk celery, chopped
1 carrot, chopped
1 teaspoon minced fresh garlic
½ cup water
3 15-ounce cans white beans (I use cannellini beans.)
1 cup vegetable broth
1 tablespoon soy sauce (I use Bragg Liquid Aminos.)
1 teaspoon dried basil
1 teaspoon dried oregano
freshly ground black pepper to taste
2 cups chopped fresh spinach

Place the onion, celery, carrot, and garlic in a large pot with the water. Cook, stirring occasionally, for 5 minutes. Add the beans, broth, soy sauce, basil, oregano, and pepper. Cook over low heat for 20 minutes. Add the spinach and cook for 3 minutes longer. Serve over grains, potatoes, toast, or English muffins.

Quick Tip: Crushing herbs releases flavor. Crush dried herbs in the palm of your hand with the fingers of your other hand. Use a mortar and pestle for hard herbs like rosemary and fennel seeds.

Disorderly Lentils
From The McDougall Quick and Easy Cookbook: Over 300 Delicious Low-Fat Recipes You Can Prepare in Fifteen Minutes or Less

Serves: 6
Preparation Time: 15 minutes
Cooking Time: 30 minutes

2 cups red lentils (I used green lentils and it turned out fine.)
4 cups water
1 onion, chopped
1 green bell pepper, chopped
½ cup grated carrot
2 cups tomato sauce
2 tablespoons soy sauce
2 tablespoons parsley flakes
1 bay leaf
½ teaspoon chopped fresh garlic
½ teaspoon basil

Combine all ingredients in a medium pot. Bring to a boil, reduce heat, cover, and simmer for 30 minutes. Serve over toast, fat-free crumpets, whole wheat English muffins, or whole wheat rolls. This recipe could also be served over baked potatoes or grains. This recipe freezes well and reheat well.

Savory Miso Broccoli + Spiced Lentil Power Plate
From Kathy Patalsky
http://kblog.lunchboxbunch.com/2013/07/savory-miso-broccoli-spiced-lentil.html

Serves 1-2

Savory Miso Broccoli:

½ teaspoon extra virgin olive oil
1 small bunch of broccoli (about 2-3 cups of chopped florets)
1 ½ tablespoons white miso paste
1 teaspoon tamari
¼ cup water
2-3 tablespoons nutritional yeast
pepper to taste
optional: a few splashes of rice vinegar, apple cider vinegar, or lemon
        juice

Toasty Spiced Lentils:

½ teaspoon extra virgin olive oil
1 can cooked lentils, drained and rinsed well
spices (any will work, Kathy just used some fine black pepper)
2 small lemons, juiced
2 tablespoons fresh flat leaf parsley, finely chopped
¼ cup white onion, diced

Tahini Sauce:

1 tablespoon tahini
1-2 teaspoons grade B maple syrup
1 tablespoon lemon juice

Other:

½ avocado, sliced
2-3 fresh orange slices
1 handful mixed greens

Open lentils and drain liquid from the can. Rinse lentils in cold water very well. Set aside.

Wash and chop your broccoli. Chop onion and parsley and juice lemons.

Whisk together your miso base for the broccoli. Add the miso, water, and tamari to a cup and stir until thinned.

Heat a large skillet over high heat. Add ½ teaspoon of olive oil. Add the broccoli and toss in the oil a bit. Add the miso-water mixture over the top of the broccoli and cover with a skillet lid. Allow the broccoli to steam and cook for about 1-2 minutes over high heat. When the broccoli is just about tender enough to serve, add in the nutritional yeast. This will coat the broccoli and add a nice extra layer of savory flavor. Add an optional splash of vinegar or lemon juice if the broccoli looks a bit too dry. You could also add in another splash of water if needed and allow that to steam the broccoli further. Cook until all the liquid has been absorbed and a nice coating coats your broccoli. Transfer hot broccoli to a serving plate.

No need to wash the skillet. Add a ½ teaspoon of olive oil and the lentils, spices, and onion. Using a spatula, scrape the sides of the pan so that any leftover "sauce" from the broccoli mingles with the lentils. Add in a splash of lemon juice to help deglaze the pan. Toast the lentils for about 1-3 minutes over high heat. Just as the lentils seem done, add in the parsley and lemon juice. Serve lentils when they are toasted and almost become "fluffy" as the outside skins toast up and the inside becomes soft from the heat.

Add your handful of greens to the plate, next to the broccoli. Then add the lentils over top. Add the avocado and citrus and a few pinches of freshly chopped parsley as well. Lastly, whisk together the tahini sauce and drizzle it over top of your plate as desired.

Serve warm and steamy.

This dish turns out to be quite savory and a bit on the salty side from all of the flavors. If you are watching your sodium or just do not like it too salty, start off using half the indicated miso. Be very aware if the lentils you are using are salted. If not, you may want to add a splash of tamari to the lentil sauté. To reduce the sodium in this dish, simply add less of the tamari and miso. You can substitute these with water, lemon juice, or vinegar.

Skillet-Popped Lentils, Harvest Skillet Style
From Kathy Patalsky,
http://kblog.lunchboxbunch.com/2013/09/skillet-popped-lentils-aka-lentils-my.html

Serves 2-3.

Skillet-Popped Lentils, Base Recipe

1 15-ounce can lentils, rinsed well in cool water and drained
fine black pepper, to taste
salt to taste (if lentils are unsalted in can)
¼ cup finely chopped parsley (a few generous pinches per cup of lentils)
1 teaspoon extra virgin olive oil (or to taste - this helps with the crispy edges while cooking)
cayenne (optional, add a pinch for extra spicy lentils)

Open your can of lentils and drain liquid. Rinse the lentils in cool water very well. Then drain all the excess water by tossing the lentils in a large bowl strainer. I use a fine mesh strainer. Fluff the lentils a bit so they are as dry as possible. Pat them dry with a paper towel if needed.

Warm a large skillet over high heat. Add ½-1 teaspoon of extra virgin olive oil. Spread around pan.

When oil is hot, add about ¾ cup of lentils. Move them through the oil a bit and let them sit there sizzling in the pan. They will start to plump up and almost look like they are about to pop. Shake the pan a bit to toss the lentils for even cooking.

After about a minute, shake about 1/8 teaspoon (or to taste) of fine black pepper over the lentils. You can also add some salt if your canned lentils were not salted (check the can). Toss the lentils with the pepper and continue cooking. You can also add in the optional cayenne if you want extra spicy lentils. You can even add other varieties of spices like chipotle powder, garlic powder, turmeric, nutritional yeast, curry powder, and onion powder.

You will know the lentils are ready when they look nutty, toasty and the edges are browned and dried. For the last minute of cooking, add in a few pinches of the chopped parsley and toss in pan to wilt with the lentils. Add more spices if desired

Remove these lentils and repeat the process with the remaining uncooked lentils.

Serve warm or cool in fridge for serving cool and adding to salads, lentil toast, and more.

Harvest Skillet Variation

½ of one small red or orange bell pepper, diced (You can use the other half to serve the lentils in.)
½ green apple, diced
¼ cup diced butternut squash or sweet potato (optional)
pinch of grated orange peel
1/8 teaspoon cinnamon
splash of apple cider vinegar
½ teaspoon extra virgin olive oil

optional: other vegetables and herbs like diced sweet onion, chopped green onion, chopped mushrooms, chopped greens like kale, and chopped sage.

Cook your lentils according to the base recipe above. Set warm cooked lentils aside.

Add a small drizzle of oil to skillet and add in the harvest vegetables and apple. Toss around in pan, adding in the spices and orange peel as well. Cook over medium-high heat until the apples and vegetables begin to brown.

Keep the vegetables in the pan and add in the cooked lentils. Toss together over medium heat. Add the splash of vinegar and continue to cook allowing the flavors of the lentils and the vegetables to mingle. This should take just a few minutes. The longer you cook, the drier your ingredients will get.

Spiced Lentils and Rice
From Susan Voisin, FatFree Vegan Kitchen
http://blog.fatfreevegan.com/2006/07/spiced-lentils-and-rice.html

Susan has asked that her recipes not be re-posted. Please follow the link above for the recipe.

If you are looking for a very rich tasting recipe, this one isn't it. This is a very simple, wholesome dish that I appreciate because of its simplicity. It's just brown rice, I use brown jasmine rice, lentils, and a few spices.

Mary McCartney's Hot Pot Recipe
From PETA Living E-News: Summer 2013 Beauty Essentials!

Serves 4

3 large or 6 medium potatoes, cut widthwise into thin round slices
3 medium onions, halved and cut widthwise into thin slices
2 medium carrots, cut into cubes
1 cup green beans, trimmed and chopped
1 15-ounce can butter beans, drained
3 vegan sausages or burgers, cooked and chipped into chunky, bite-
    sized pieces (optional)
2 tablespoons chopped fresh parsley or 2 teaspoons dried mixed herbs
3 1/3 cups vegetable stock (allowed to cool) mixed with 1 tablespoon
    corn starch
2 tablespoons light olive oil (I used 1 tablespoon and it was fine.)
Black pepper, to taste

Preheat the oven to 350 degrees F.

Talk half the potato slices and arrange them in the bottom of a
casserole or baking dish (approximately 11 inches). Top with the
onion slices, spreading evenly, followed by the carrots and green beans,
the butter beans, and the sausage or burger pieces. Sprinkle with the
parsley and finish with a layer of the remaining potato slices.

Carefully pour in the vegetable stock, which should come to about 3/8
of an inch below the top layer of potato slices. Drizzle with the olive
oil, season with the black pepper, and cover with baking foil.

Place on the middle shelf in the oven and cook for 1 hour and 45
minutes.

Remove the baking foil, dot the potatoes with vegan margarine or olive
oil, and cook until the top layer of potatoes is golden and slightly crisp,
about 15 minutes more.

Menestra
From Moosewood Restaurant Cooks at Home

Serves 4

1-2 onions (1 ½ - 2 cups sliced)
3 garlic cloves (I use more.)
2 medium carrots (about 1 ½ cups sliced)
1 large potato (about 2 cups diced)
1 tablespoon sweet paprika (I use more.)
2 bay leaves
pinch of cayenne (I use more.)
2 cups hot water *
½ cup dry sherry (I use ¾ cup.)
½ teaspoon salt
½ pound mushrooms
1 red bell pepper
5 artichokes (1 14-ounce can packed in water)
1 cup fresh or frozen peas
salt to taste
chopped Spanish olives (optional)

Halve and thinly slice the onion, then cut the slices in half. Mince or press the garlic. In a pot, sauté the onions and garlic in a small amount of water on medium heat until tender adding water as necessary to keep the food from sticking. Cut the carrots in half lengthwise, then slice them crosswise into half circles, and add them to the pot. Cut the potato into ½ - inch cubes. Add the potato, paprika, bay leaves, and cayenne and sauté for a minute or so, stirring to prevent sticking. Pour in the water, sherry, and salt. Cover the pot and bring to a boil. Reduce the heat to a simmer.

Wash the mushrooms and cut off and discard the stems. Leave any small mushrooms whole, but cut the larger ones into halves or quarters. Chop the pepper into 1-inch pieces. Add the mushrooms and peppers to the pot. Cut the artichoke hearts into halves. When the vegetables are just tender, stir in the artichokes and peas. Simmer for 3 to 4 minutes. Add salt to taste.

Serve with chopped olives if you like.

* or use the liquid from the canned artichoke hearts plus enough water to make a total of 2 cups.

Roasted Ratatouille
From Moosewood Restaurant Simple Suppers

Makes 4 servings.

1 zucchini
3 onions
1 eggplant, peeled
2 tomatoes
2 red, green, or yellow bell peppers
6 garlic cloves
1-2 tablespoons olive oil
1 teaspoon salt
½ teaspoon black pepper
1 cup packed fresh basil leaves

Preheat the oven to 450 degrees F.

Cut all of the vegetables into 1-inch chunks and place them in a large bowl. You need between 12 and 14 cups total. Coarsely chop the garlic. Toss the vegetables and garlic with the olive oil, salt, pepper, and spread on two baking sheets. Roast for 15 minutes, then stir the vegetables. Continue to roast for 25 to 30 minutes, stirring again after 20 minutes, until the vegetables are fork-tender and juicy.

While the vegetables roast, chop the basil. When the vegetables are done, put them in a serving bowl and stir in the chopped basil.

Vegan Macaroni and Cheese
From Katherine Lawrence

Makes 10 cups.

4 cups dry whole wheat elbow macaroni or shell pasta
2 cups non-dairy milk, unflavored
1 cup vegetable broth
¾ cup nutritional yeast (a great source of protein and B vitamins)
¾ teaspoon salt
½ teaspoon dry mustard
½ teaspoon ground black pepper
¼ teaspoon paprika
1/8 teaspoon garlic powder
1/16 teaspoon turmeric
¼ cup whole wheat flour

Prepare pasta according to package directions. Set aside.

In a small saucepan, simmer on medium-high heat all ingredients with the exception of the flour until hot and bubbling. Whisk in flour and heat until there are no more lumps and the mixture is bubbling and thick.

Add to pasta, mix, and enjoy. This is a delicious dish that is cholesterol free and low in fat.

There are approximately 242 calories per cup.

Chipotle Mac and "Cheese" with Roasted Brussels Sprouts
From People for the Ethical Treatment of Animals

Serves 4

1 pound Brussels sprouts, quartered
1 tablespoon olive oil
dash of salt, plus more for seasoning
1 cup cashews, soaked in water for at least 2 hours
4 chipotles, seeded (I could only find these in a can mixed with adobo
        sauce. I rinsed the sauce off of them prior to using.)
1 cup vegetable broth
2 cloves garlic
2 tablespoons nutritional yeast flakes
2 tablespoons miso
8 ounces macaroni, any type

Preheat oven to 425 degrees F.

Line a large baking sheet with parchment paper. Toss the quartered Brussels sprouts with the olive oil and a dash of salt. Bake for 18 minutes, or until lightly browned.

Put the drained cashews, chipotles, vegetable broth, garlic, nutritional yeast flakes, and miso in a blender and blend until completely smooth.

Cook the pasta according to the package directions. Drain the noodles and place immediately back in the pot on low heat.

Add the chipotle sauce and stir for a few minutes until the sauce thickens and everything is creamy.

Season with salt, if needed, and stir in the Brussels sprouts. Serve.

Cheesy Cauliflower Sauce
From Susan Voisin, FatFree Vegan Kitchen
http://blog.fatfreevegan.com/2013/05/cheesy-cauliflower-sauce.html

Susan has asked that her recipes not be re-posted. Please follow the link above for the recipe.

Cheezy Sauce
Skinny Bitch in the Kitch by Rory Freedman and Kim Barnouin

Makes about 2 ¾ cups.

About 2 cups soy or rice milk
¼ cup refined coconut oil
¼ cup whole wheat pastry flour (I use whole wheat flour and it turns
    out fine.)
8 ounces vegan cheese (cheddar, mozzarella, Jack, whatever you like, or
    a combination), shredded (I use Daiya cheese.)
½ teaspoon fine sea salt
¼ teaspoon white pepper (I use black pepper.)

In a 1-quart saucepan over low heat, heat 2 cups of soy or rice milk
until it's barely simmering (small bubbles will appear at the edges of the
pan). Cover and set aside.

Heat the oil in a 2- to 3-quart saucepan over medium heat. Whisk in
the flour and cook, whisking constantly, for 2 minutes. Slowly whisk in
the hot milk and bring the mixture to a simmer. Reduce heat to low
and cook, whisking often, until the sauce is thick and no longer tastes
of raw flour, 6 to 8 minutes. Remove from heat and whisk in the
cheese, salt, and pepper, stirring until cheese melts (if necessary, return
the pot to low heat). If not using immediately, transfer the sauce to a
bowl, cover with plastic wrap directly on the surface of the sauce, and
use within 30 minutes. If the sauce gets too thick while it sits, whisk in
a little more warm soy or rice milk.

No-Meat Loaf
From The Cancer Survivor's Guide by Neal D. Barnard, MD and Jennifer K. Reilly, RD

Serves 12.

14 ounces vegan burger crumbles (Beyond Meat for example)
1 ½ cups bread crumbs, preferably whole wheat
1 ¼ cups rolled oats
1 cup tomato sauce or crushed tomatoes
1 small onion, minced
2 celery stalks, minced
1 carrot, minced
½ green bell pepper, minced
¼ cup finely chopped walnuts
3 tablespoons reduced-sodium soy sauce (I use Bragg's Amino Acids)
2 teaspoons stone-ground or Dijon mustard
½ teaspoon dried thyme
½ teaspoon dried sage
¼ teaspoon ground black pepper
½ cup ketchup or barbeque sauce (optional)

Preheat oven to 350 degrees F. Lightly mist a 5"x9" loaf pan or similar baking dish with vegetable oil spray.

Combine the vegan burger crumbles, bread crumbs, oats, tomato sauce, onion, celery, carrot, bell pepper, walnuts, soy sauce, mustard, thyme, sage, and pepper in a large bowl. Mix with a large spoon or your hands until the mixture is evenly combined.

Press into the prepared loaf pan. Spread the optional ketchup over the top and bake for 60 minutes. Let stand for 10 minutes before slicing.

To store leftovers, remove the loaf from the pan and let cool. Stored in a covered container in the refrigerator, leftover No-Meat Loaf will keep for up to 3 days.

Per serving: 104 calories; 2.6 g fat; 0.3 g saturated fat; 22% calories from fat; 0 mg cholesterol; 8.2 g protein; 13.9 g carbohydrate; 2.7 g sugar; 2.5 g fiber; 418 mg sodium; 37 mg calcium; 1.7 mg iron; 5.9 mg vitamin C; 463 mcg beta-carotene; 0.6 mg vitamin E; 3094 mcg lycopene

Polenta with Black Beans and Mango Salsa
From The Starch Solution

Serves 6 to 8

Preparation Time: 15 minutes
Cooking Time: 20 minutes

1 package (24 ounces) cooked polenta, cut into ½"-thick slices
½ cup vegetable broth
1 onion, chopped
1 red bell pepper, chopped
1 orange or yellow bell pepper, chopped
2 cloves garlic, crushed or minced
2 cans (15 ounces each) black beans, drained and rinsed
1 can (15 ounces) crushed tomatoes (I used fire roasted and it added a
    lot of flavor)
1 can (4 ounces) chopped green chilies
1 teaspoon chili powder
1 teaspoon ground cumin
Dash or two of Tabasco or other hot sauce
Freshly ground black pepper
¼ cup chopped fresh cilantro
2 cups store-bought mango salsa

Preheat oven to 375 degrees F. Place the polenta slices on a nonstick baking sheet and bake for 15 minutes (I made polenta from a box, did not slice or bake it, and it tasted fine).

While the polenta bakes, put the broth, onion, bell peppers, and garlic in a large saucepan. Cook, stirring occasionally, until the vegetables soften, about 5 minutes. Add the black beans, tomatoes, chilies, chili powder, cumin, hot sauce, and black pepper to taste. Cook 10 minutes. Taste and add more hot sauce if you wish. Stir in the cilantro and remove the saucepan from the heat.

To serve, arrange a few slices of polenta on each plate and top with the black bean mixture. Top with the mango salsa or serve it in a bowl on the side.

Tofu Nuggets
From Betty Crocker Easy Vegetarian

Children love this recipe!

Makes 4 or 5 servings.

3 tablespoons all-purpose flour
6 tablespoons cold water
2/3 cup vegan dry bread crumbs
1 teaspoon salt
1 14-ounce package firm tofu, drained and cut into 1-inch cubes
vegetable oil
barbeque sauce, sweet and sour sauce, or ketchup

Beat flour and water with wire whisk or hand beater until smooth.

Toss bread crumbs and salt in bowl or pie plate. Add other seasonings such as a dash of cayenne pepper and black pepper.

Dip tofu cubes into batter, then roll all sides in bread crumbs to coat.

Heat a scant amount of oil in a skillet over medium-high heat. Cook about one minute on each side until golden brown.

Serve with your choice of sauce(s).

Spicy Kale
From Moosewood Restaurant Cooks at Home

Serves 4

1 large onion, diced (about 1 ½ cups)
1-1 ½ teaspoons oil
1 bunch kale (about 2 pounds)
2 teaspoons vinegar (or to taste)
¼ teaspoon crushed red pepper flakes (or more to taste)
salt and ground black pepper to taste

Sauté the onion in the oil in a large skillet, saucepan, or wok on low heat for about 10 minutes, until translucent. While the onion sautés, thoroughly rinse the kale. Remove and coarsely chop the leaves and discard the large stems.

Add the moist kale to the onions and cook, covered, for about 5 minutes, stirring occasionally, until the leaves are wilted but still bright green. Stir in the vinegar and red pepper flakes. Add salt and pepper to taste, and serve immediately or at room temperature.

Braised Mixed Vegetables
From Tracey Eakin

You can braise almost any vegetable. I braise as many vegetables as will fit in my largest skillet in just enough water to keep the vegetables from sticking, adding additional water as needed. I start with the vegetables that need a longer time in the skillet to cook such as onions, purple cabbage, and Brussels sprouts, and add in later, vegetables that cook faster like spinach. I season with minced garlic, salt, pepper, and a little cayenne pepper or crushed red pepper flakes if I want a little heat. About halfway through the cooking process, I add ½ tablespoon of olive oil. I try to keep added oils to a minimum and continue to strive to add less every time I make a dish. Pictured above are chopped onion, shredded purple cabbage, halved Brussels sprouts, mushroom slices, chopped asparagus, spinach, and chopped yellow bell peppers. Cook until the vegetables are tender but still a little crisp and brightly colored. Cooking them too long will result in mushy vegetables.

Simple Bean and Vegetable Braise
From Tracey Eakin

onion
mushrooms
asparagus
beans

Sure-Fire Roasted Vegetables
From The Cancer Survivor's Guide by Neal D. Barnard, MD and Jennifer K. Reilly, RD

Mixed Vegetable Combo:
1 cup chopped broccoli florets
1 cup diced onion
1 cup diced bell peppers
1 cup diced zucchini or yellow squash
1 cup diced eggplant
1-3 garlic cloves, minced or pressed
1/3 cup Italian, Mexican, or Indian Seasoning Mix
1 ½ cups cooked or canned chickpeas or black beans, rinsed and drained

Root Vegetable Combo:
1 cup chopped carrots
1 cup chopped sweet potatoes or new potatoes
1 cup peeled and chopped butternut or other winter squash
1 cup peeled and chopped parsnips or rutabaga
1 cup chopped onion
1-3 garlic cloves, minced or pressed
1/3 cup Italian, Mexican, or Indian Seasoning Mix
1 ½ cups cooked or canned chickpeas or black beans, rinsed and drained

Italian Seasoning Mix:
¼ cup chopped fresh parsley
2 teaspoons dried basil
2 teaspoons dried rosemary
1 teaspoon dried oregano
¼ teaspoon salt
¼ teaspoon ground black pepper

Combine all of the ingredients in a small bowl.

Mexican Seasoning Mix:
¼ cup minced fresh cilantro
2 teaspoons ground cumin

1 teaspoon dried basil
1 teaspoon dried rosemary
¼ teaspoon salt
¼ teaspoon ground black pepper

Combine all of the ingredients in a small bowl.

India Seasoning Mix:
¼ cup minced fresh cilantro
1 teaspoon curry powder
1 teaspoon garam masala
¼ teaspoon salt
¼ teaspoon ground black pepper

Combine all of the ingredients in a small bowl.

Preheat oven to 400 degrees F. Lightly mist a large, shallow baking pan (such as a jelly roll pan) with vegetable oil spray.

Select one of the vegetable combos and place the prepared vegetables in a large bowl. Add your choice of seasoning mix and toss until the vegetables are evenly coated. Transfer to the prepared baking pan and spread out in a single layer.

Roast in the oven for ten minutes. Remove the pan from the oven and mist the top of the vegetables lightly with the vegetable oil spray. Turn the vegetables over and roast for 5-10 minutes longer (root vegetables could take up to 30 minutes longer), or until they are evenly tender.

Stir in the beans and serve hot from the oven.

Stored in a covered container in the refrigerator, leftover Sure-Fire Roasted Vegetables will keep for up to two days.

Easy Roasted Beets
From Susan Voisin
http://blog.fatfreevegan.com/2006/09/puy-lentil-salad-with-roasted-beets.html?wptouch_preview_theme=enabled

Wash and scrub beets well. Wrap each beet (first in parchment paper, then) in aluminum foil and bake at 350 degrees F for about an hour (I did this in the toaster oven with 2 beets, and it worked well.). Allow the beets to cool, then peel them and slice or dice them.

Special Holiday Recipes

Thanksgiving Day Special: Bread and Herb Casserole
From Ecological Cooking: Recipes to Save the Planet

This is my favorite Thanksgiving casserole. It is a fabulous replacement for traditional stuffing.

Serves 4

4 cups whole grain bread cubes (recipe below)
¼ teaspoon sage
¼ teaspoon thyme
¼ teaspoon rosemary, crushed
¼ teaspoon marjoram
1 tablespoon dried parsley
1 tablespoon nutritional yeast
salt and freshly ground black pepper, to taste
½ cup chopped onion
3 tablespoons olive oil (I use 1 tablespoon and it turns out just fine.)
½ cup lightly chopped walnuts
½ cup chopped celery
½ cup sliced mushrooms
½ cup chopped dried fruit (I use a blend of dried cranberries, raisins, and golden raisins.)
2 tablespoons tamari (I use Bragg Liquid Aminos, a healthy alternative to soy sauce, available in most grocery and health food stores.)
½ cup boiling water or vegetable stock

Preheat oven to 350 degrees F.

Mix bread cubes with herbs, nutritional yeast, salt, and pepper. Add onions, oil, walnuts, celery, mushrooms, and fruit. Combine tamari and boiling water or stock, and pour all over to moisten, adding more liquid if mixture is too dry. Place in a lightly oiled 1-quart baking dish (I do not oil it and it is just fine.), cover, and bake for 20 minutes. Uncover and bake for 10 minutes longer. Serve with your favorite vegan gravy or mushroom sauce.

Whole grain bread cubes are very simple to make. Just cube your favorite whole grain bread (I like to use Ezekiel 4:9 Sprouted 100%

Whole Grain Bread).   Place on cookie sheets and bake for 15-20 minutes at 350 degrees F until dry but not browned. Let cool before using.

Vegan Green Bean Casserole
From Susan Voisin, FatFree Vegan Kitchen

http://blog.fatfreevegan.com/2006/11/best-vegan-green-bean-casserole.html

Susan has asked that her recipes not be re-posted. Please follow the link above for the recipe.

Yam and Apple Casserole
From Karen Shanahan, Avani Institute, http://avani-institute.com/

4 large yams
3 large cooking apples
3 tablespoons Earth Balance buttery spread
1 tablespoon cornstarch or arrowroot powder
½ cup firmly packed brown sugar
1 tablespoon fresh lemon juice
2 cups hot apple juice
½ teaspoon allspice
½ teaspoon cinnamon
½ cup raisins

Preheat oven to 350 degrees F.

Boil yams for 30 minutes. Peel and slice 1/3 inch thick.

Peel, core, and thinly slice apples.

In a small saucepan, melt buttery spread. Add cornstarch, brown sugar, lemon juice, hot apple juice, and spices. Cook 6 minutes.

In a 9"x13" casserole dish, alternate layers of yam and apple slices. Sprinkle raisins on top. Pour the hot mixture over the yams, apples, and raisins. Cover with parchment paper and then with foil and bake for one hour. Remove the parchment paper and foil and bake for an additional 15 minutes.

New Year's Day Special: Mashed Potatoes, Sauerkraut, and Green Beans
From Tracey Eakin Using Her Aunt Karen's Sauerkraut Recipe

Mashed Potatoes:

Scrub potatoes and cut into chunks. Cook in boiling water until tender. Drain and blend with unsweetened non-dairy milk until it reaches the desired consistency. Salt and pepper to taste.

Sauerkraut:

Makes approximately 2 large servings.

27 ounces of sauerkraut
½ cup filtered water
1 small onion, chopped
1 Granny Smith apple, skinned and chopped
¼ cup ketchup
1 tablespoon dark brown sugar
½ tablespoon caraway seeds
1 tablespoon Earth Balance buttery spread

Combine and simmer for two hours.

Green Beans:

Steam freshly cleaned green beans.

Pressure Cooker Recipes

Mushroom Chili
From Chef AJ
Adapted from The Low Fat Herbivore by Jocelyn Graef
https://www.youtube.com/watch?v=7jsAVBCQfYg

2 pounds crimini mushrooms, washed and sliced (I use portabella
      mushrooms.)
10 ounces pre-cut onions
8 cloves garlic, put through a press
2 cans salt-free, fire-roasted tomatoes
1 can salt-free pinto beans
1 can salt-free kidney beans
1 can salt-free black beans
1 teaspoon dry mustard powder
1 teaspoon crushed red pepper flakes
½ teaspoon thyme
½ teaspoon oregano

Place all ingredients in an electric pressure cooker. Cook on high
pressure for 6 minutes. Release pressure. Stir in 1 pounds organic
frozen corn. Delicious served over brown rice or baked Yukon gold
potato.

This recipe reminds me more of a soup or stew and less of a chili, but
it is delicious nonetheless.

Salad Dressings

Low-Fat Tahini-Chickpea Dressing
From Susan Voisin, FatFree Vegan Kitchen

http://blog.fatfreevegan.com/2011/08/low-fat-tahini-chickpea-dressing.html

Susan has asked that her recipes not be re-posted. Please follow the link above for the recipe.

This dressing is wonderful with greens like the kale pictured below as the fat in the tahini increases the kale phytonutrients' bioavailability. Raw nuts and seeds will accomplish the same thing.

Artichoke Brazil Nut Dressing
From Unprocessed by Chef AJ

½ cup raw Brazil nuts
1 14-ounce can water-packed artichoke hearts, rinsed and drained
1 cup unsweetened almond milk
¼ cup fresh lemon juice
¼ cup rice vinegar
4 tablespoons nutritional yeast
1 teaspoon salt-free seasoning, or more to taste (I use 3 teaspoons of
     Mrs. Dash Garlic & Herb Blend.)

Grind the Brazil nuts in your blender or in a coffee grinder. Place remaining ingredients in the blender along with the nuts and blend until smooth and creamy (I also add some black pepper.).

Hidden Cashew Ranch Dressing
From Susan Voisin, FatFree Vegan Kitchen

http://blog.fatfreevegan.com/2012/01/hidden-cashew-ranch-dressing-plus-tips-for-eating-salads-when-you-really-dont-want-to.html

Susan has asked that her recipes not be re-posted. Please follow the link above for the recipe.

Drizzle this dressing over hot pasta for a delicious Alfredo-like sauce.

Snacks/Desserts

Broccoli and Peanut Dip
From Food to Go with Steph and Ro on YouTube.com
http://www.youtube.com/watch?v=xL0lg95GopQ

Fresh or frozen broccoli florets
2 tablespoons creamy peanut butter
2 tablespoons Bragg Liquid Aminos (soy sauce can be used instead)
2 tablespoons seasoned rice vinegar
¼ teaspoon minced garlic
1 teaspoon agave nectar
1/8 teaspoon powdered ginger

Steam broccoli florets. Mix peanut butter, liquid aminos, seasoned rice vinegar, garlic, agave nectar, and ginger. Can be used as a dip for the broccoli florets or to top baked potatoes, rice, noodles, or pasta.

"Ranch" Dip
From People for the Ethical Treatment of Animals

Mix Tofutti Sour Supreme Better Than Sour Cream vegan sour cream with Knorr's Vegetable recipe mix. I use a little more than ½ cup of the vegan sour cream with one 1.4-ounce packet of seasoning mix. Adjust to your tastes and pick your favorite vegetables to dip.

Roasted Chickpeas with Red Chili Pepper Flakes
From People for the Ethical Treatment of Animals

Serves 4.

1 15-ounce can chickpeas (garbanzo beans), drained and rinsed
1 teaspoon extra virgin olive oil
1 teaspoon fresh black pepper
1 teaspoon sea salt
½ teaspoon cumin
½ teaspoon paprika
1 tablespoon red chili pepper flakes

Preheat oven to 400 degrees F.

Pat the chickpeas dry with a paper towel. Discard any skins that peel off.

Combine the remaining ingredients in a small bowl and add the chickpeas. Stir until the beans are evenly coated.

Place on a baking sheet and roast for 30 to 40 minutes, turning once.

Serve immediately.

I love this recipe but I back off the spices a little when I make it. Feel free to adjust accordingly to your tastes.

Microwave Potato Chips

I've purchased two different microwave potato chip makers at Bed, Bath & Beyond. The first one had the potato chips placed vertically on a plastic rack. When I microwaved the potato chips too long, the plastic rack melted. Not good! The second one contained a rubber tray. This one worked well. I used a mandolin and carefully sliced up a clean potato with the skins intact. I microwaved them in batches on this tray in a single layer for 3-3½ minutes each batch.

If you prefer not to have to purchase a kit, you can place your potato chips directly on parchment paper. Complete directions can be found at the following link:

http://blog.fatfreevegan.com/2008/08/healthy-crunchy-three-guilt-free-snacks.html

Just scroll down the page to the potato chips.

Oatmeal Goji Berry Balls
From The Cancer Project Food for Life Weekly Recipe

Makes 3 dozen.

2 ½ cups rolled oats or quinoa flakes (I use rolled oats.)
3 medium ripe bananas
1/3 cup raw almonds or walnuts, ground in a food processor until they
        become coarse crumbs
1 cup chopped, pitted dates (chopped to same size as goji berries)
1 cup goji berries, soaked for 15 minutes in warm water, then drained
        (can be found in most health food stores)
½ teaspoon sea salt or Himalayan salt
1 tablespoon vanilla extract

Preheat oven to 325 degrees F. Line a cookie sheet with unbleached parchment paper.

Place oats or quinoa flakes in a blender or a food processor and pulse on and off until oats/quinoa flakes turn into coarse crumbs/flour.

In a medium bowl, mash bananas with a fork. Add ground almonds or walnuts, dates, and drained goji berries. Mix well. Add salt, vanilla, and ground oats or quinoa flakes and stir well to combine.

Use wet hands or form tablespoon-size balls. Place on parchment-lined cookie sheet and bake for 25 minutes, rotating pan halfway through bake time.

Per two balls: 110 calories; 2.2 g fat; 0.2 g saturated fat; 16.5% calories from fat; 0 mg cholesterol; 20.9 g carbohydrate; 3.1 g fiber; 8.5 g sugar; 2.9 g protein; 66 mg sodium; 2 mg vitamin C; 47 mcg beta-carotene; 0.8 mg vitamin E; 18 mg calcium; 0.8 mg iron

Energy Balls
From Uma Purighalla, MD
http://theplantbasedplate.com/20501.html

Makes about 20 small, plum-sized balls.

1 cup almonds, soaked overnight
1 1/3 cups pitted dates, soaked in warm water for at least 5 minutes
¾ cup dried, grated, unsweetened coconut
1-2 teaspoons cinnamon (or 1-2 teaspoons cardamom powder for an
    Indian version)

Drain the almonds and the dates and place them in a food processor.
Add the coconut and vanilla or cardamom. Blend well and roll into
balls.

Chewy, Homemade Granola Bars
From Wendy Irene

Makes 12 large bars

½ cup cashews, raw and unsalted
4 cups old fashioned oatmeal
½ cup dried cranberries
½ teaspoon cinnamon
½ cup semi-sweet, dairy-free chocolate chips
3 tablespoons ground flax seed
1 cup peanut butter
1/3 cup brown rice syrup
½ cup brown sugar
1 vanilla bean or 1 teaspoon pure vanilla extract
1 ripe banana, mashed

Preheat oven to 350 degrees F. Spread raw cashews on a baking sheet and bake for 8 minutes. Allow to cool. When the cashews are cooled, chop into smaller pieces.

In a large mixing bowl, combine dry ingredients - cashew pieces, oats, cranberries, cinnamon, chocolate chips, and ground flax seed. Stir and set aside.

Using a paring knife, carefully slice the vanilla bean in half lengthwise. Using the back of the knife, gently run it along the inside of the vanilla bean scraping the seeds out. Repeat for the other half of the vanilla bean. Alternatively, you can use 1 teaspoon of pure vanilla extract.

In a medium saucepan over low heat, add the vanilla bean seeds or pure vanilla extract, peanut butter, brown rice syrup, brown sugar, and mashed banana. Stir for a few minutes until melted and mixed together.

Add the peanut butter mixture to the large mixing bowl with oats. Stir until everything is evenly coated.

Place the granola mixture into a square silicon brownie pan or 9"x13" pan. If you do not have a silicon pan, line the pan with parchment paper prior to placing the mixture in the pan. Press down firmly with the back of a spoon, the back of a measuring cup, or using a piece of parchment paper on top of the mixture, press it into the pan with your hands.

Refrigerate for 50 minutes, then freeze for 10 minutes before cutting into bars and removing from the pan. If using a silicon pan, you may want to remove the mixture prior to cutting into bars so as not to damage the pan.

The bars will keep in an airtight container in the refrigerator for up to a week and can probably be frozen.

Apple Cranberry Crisp
From The Cancer Project Food for Life Weekly Recipe

Makes 8 servings.

2 large, tart apples, peeled and sliced
½ cup fresh or frozen cranberries (I couldn't find these so I used plenty of frozen, whole cherries.)
¾ cup Grape-Nuts cereal or any high fiber whole wheat cereal
¾ cup rolled oats
½ teaspoon cinnamon
1/3 cup brown rice syrup (Sometimes I use agave nectar.)
2/3 cup apple juice
¼ teaspoon cornstarch or arrowroot

Preheat oven to 350 degrees F.

Arrange apple slices in a 9"x9" baking dish, then sprinkle with cranberries.

In a bowl, mix cereal, oats, and cinnamon, then stir in brown rice syrup. Spread evenly over apples.

In a small bowl or measuring cup, mix apple juice and cornstarch or arrowroot, then pour evenly over other ingredients.

Bake for 50 minutes, or until apples are tender (I bake it covered for 40 minutes, then uncovered for 10 minutes, so that the topping crisps, but making sure the topping doesn't burn.).

Per 1/8 of the recipe: 148 calories; 0.9 g fat; 0.2 g saturated fat; 5.3% calories from fat; 0 mg cholesterol; 35.1 g carbohydrate; 3 g fiber; 14.4 g sugar; 2.5 g protein; 84 mg sodium; 3 mg vitamin C; 20 mcg beta-carotene; 0.2 mg vitamin E; 14 mg calcium; 3.5 mg iron

Oatmeal Banana Bites
From Jill Eckart, CHHC, Physicians Committee for Responsible Medicine's Food for Life Recipe of the Week

Makes 8 to 10 servings

1 cup rolled oats
1 cup oat flour
1 teaspoon baking powder
¼ teaspoon sea salt
½ teaspoon cinnamon
1/8 - ¼ teaspoon freshly ground nutmeg (I use ¼ teaspoon ground
    nutmeg.)
1 cup pureed overripe bananas (roughly 2 large bananas, see note)
1 teaspoon vanilla extract
2 tablespoons grain-sweetened vegan chocolate chips or raisins (op
    tional) (I use 1 tablespoon of each.)

Preheat oven to 350 degrees F. In a mixing bowl, combine the oats, oat flour, baking powder, sea salt, cinnamon, and nutmeg. Stir well until combined. Add the pureed banana and vanilla (and chocolate chips or raisins, if using) to the dry mixture, and stir until combined. Using a cookie scoop or spoon, place mounds of the batter (about 2 to 2 ½ tablespoons) on to a baking sheet lined with parchment paper. Bake for 14 to 15 minutes, until golden and set to the touch. Remove and let cool on pan for just a minute, then transfer to a cooling rack.

Note: Use an immersion blender and a deep cup to puree your bananas (this is the easiest, but a blender or small food processor also works). It produces a very liquefied mixture, not like what you can get through mashing.

Per serving (1 muffin): 114 calories, 2 g fat, 0.3 g saturated fat, 12% calories from fat, 0 mg cholesterol, 3 g protein, 22 g carbohydrate, 4 g sugar, 3 g fiber, 136 mg sodium, 49 mg calcium, 1 mg iron, 2 mg vitamin C, 8 mcg beta-carotene, 0.1 mg vitamin E

Banana-Maple Oatmeal Cookies
From Susan Voisin, FatFree Vegan Kitchen
http://blog.fatfreevegan.com/2010/02/banana-maple-oatmeal-cookies.html

Makes 18 cookies.

1 teaspoon ground chia seeds, 2 teaspoons egg replacer powder, or 2 teaspoons ground flax seed (I use the flax seed.)
2 tablespoons water
1 cup regular or quick oats (I use regular oats.)
1 cup whole wheat flour
½ teaspoon baking soda
½ teaspoon baking powder
½ teaspoon salt
1 teaspoon cinnamon
¼ cup raisins
½ teaspoon vanilla
½ cup maple syrup
1 banana, mashed
½ teaspoon lemon juice

Preheat the oven to 375 degrees F.

In a small bowl, combine the chia seeds (or egg replacer or flax seed) with the water and set aside until thickened (no waiting time is necessary if packaged egg replacer is used.).

Mix the oats, flour, baking soda, baking powder, salt, and cinnamon in a medium mixing bowl. Add the raisins.

Add the maple syrup, vanilla, mashed banana, and lemon juice to the chia/flax/egg replacer and combine well. Pour into the dry mixture and stir well but don't over mix.

Drop by heaping tablespoons onto a baking sheet lined with a silicon mat or parchment paper. Flatten each cookie slightly with a fork. Bake for 8-12 minutes or until bottoms and sides are lightly brown. Cool for a few minutes on a wire rack before serving.

Because they contain no fat, these cookies are softer the day they are made and chewier the next day. If you prefer them soft, warm your day-old cookies in the microwave for a few seconds.

Nutrition (per cookie): 78 calories, 5 calories from fat, less than 1 g total fat, 0 mg cholesterol, 115 mg sodium, 106.1 mg potassium, 17.5 g carbohydrates, 1.7 g fiber, 7.6 g sugar, 1.7 g protein, 1.3 points

Adonis Cake
From Rip Esselstyn

This cake is very good. However, it is not as light and fluffy as a store bought cake. It is a little denser, but still tastes very good. The frosting ran off the sides of the cake and onto the plate while I was icing it, but firmed up nicely later on. It would probably ice much nicer if it sat for a short while after being prepared, but not in the refrigerator, before being used.

To create a double layer cake like the one pictured above, just double the recipes below.

Cake Preparation Time: 10 minutes
Cake Cooking Time: 30 minutes

Makes 1 9"x9" cake.

Cake Ingredients:

1 ½ cups whole wheat flour
3 tablespoons unsweetened cocoa powder
1 teaspoon baking soda
2/3 cup pure maple syrup
6 tablespoons unsweetened applesauce
1 tablespoon white vinegar
1 teaspoon vanilla extract
¾ cold water

Frosting Preparation Time: 5 minutes

Makes about 2 cups of frosting.

Frosting Ingredients:

1 12-ounce package of silken tofu
¾ cup dairy-free, semi-sweet chocolate chips, melted
1 tablespoon vanilla extract
cayenne pepper (optional)

Preheat oven to 350 degrees F. Set out 9"x9" nonstick cake pan. In a mixing bowl, combine the flour, cocoa, and baking soda and mix well. Add the maple syrup, applesauce, vinegar, vanilla, and water and mix well to combine.

Pour the batter into the cake pan. Bake for 30 minutes. When the cake is done, remove it from the oven and set aside to cool. When cooled, frost.

While the cake is baking, make the Adonis frosting. Place the silken tofu in a food processor. Add the melted chocolate chips and blend. Add the vanilla and blend again until chocolaty and creamy. Taste it. If you are using grain-sweetened chips, you may want to add a bit more maple syrup. For a sweet and spicy frosting, try adding a pinch of cayenne pepper. Use immediately or refrigerate until ready to use.

This frosting can be used as a pudding as well. After preparing it, pour it into glasses, layered with sliced fruit, and refrigerate until ready to serve.

Vegan Double-Layer Pumpkin Cheesecake
From Susan Voisin, FatFree Vegan Kitchen
http://blog.fatfreevegan.com/2007/11/double-layer-pumpkin-cheesecake.html

Susan has asked that her recipes not be re-posted. Please follow the link above for the recipe.

Raw Carrot Cake with Vanilla Cream Frosting
From Christine Roseberry

http://justglowingwithhealth.com/no-bake-gluten-freecarrot-cake/

For the carrot cake:

2 cups carrot pulp (about 3-4 whole carrots, if using whole carrots, cut
        into medium chunks before placing in the food processor)
½ cup pecans, soaked for 6+ hours, drained and rinsed
1 cup Medjool dates, pitted (about 10 dates)
½ cup unsweetened, shredded coconut
1 Fuji apple, cored and cut into medium-sized pieces
1 quarter-sized chunk of ginger
½ teaspoon pure vanilla extract
½ teaspoon cinnamon

For the frosting:

1 ¼ cup cashews, soaked for 6+ hours, drained and rinsed
½ teaspoon vanilla powder (I found this at Uncommon Market in Up-
        per St. Clair.)
1 tablespoon + 2 teaspoons lemon juice (about 1 lemon)
3 Medjool dates, pitted
1/3 cup water, more or less, for desired consistency

For the cake:

Place the chunks of apple into the food processor. Blend until it
becomes coarsely shredded, being careful not to over process. The
apple should be in coarse pieces. Then add the whole carrot pieces, if
using, and pulse into coarse pieces. If using carrot pulp, add it and the
remaining ingredients and pulse until it becomes a coarse, sticky mix,
making sure not to over process.

Author's Note: To ensure that the apple and whole carrot pieces did
not get over processed, I placed them in a mixing bowl once they were
shredded. I then added the remaining cake ingredients and pulsed
them until they became a coarse, sticky mix. I also added them to the
bowl and mixed thoroughly.

Line an 8"x8" glass baking dish with parchment paper. Press the cake mixture into the dish evenly.

For the frosting:

In a high-speed blender, blend all of the frosting ingredients, except for the water. Add just enough water in small increments to make the mixture creamy. If you are using a Vitamix, you will probably have to scrape down the sides several times with a spatula. It may take up to five minutes to get it blended.

Add the frosting to the top of the cake.

Place it in freezer for about one hour, then place it in the refrigerator. Take it out of the refrigerator and let it sit for about 25 minutes before eating. Sprinkle cinnamon on top and serve.

Mocha Mousse
From The Cancer Project Food for Life Weekly Recipe

Makes 5 servings.

1 12.3-ounce package of firm silken tofu
2 tablespoons cocoa or carob powder (I use cocoa powder.)
1 tablespoon grain-based coffee substitute granules (optional, I couldn't
        find so I didn't use)
½ teaspoon vanilla extract
½ cup chopped dates or 1/3 cup date sugar * (I used chopped dates.)

Mix tofu, cocoa or carob powder, coffee substitute, if using, and vanilla
in blender. Add dates or date sugar to blender and blend thoroughly.
Chill and eat.

* Date sugar is simply made from finely ground dehydrated dates and
can be found in most health food stores.

Per 1/3 cup serving: 97 calories; 2.3 g fat; 0.5 g saturated fat; 20.9%
calories from fat; 5.7 g protein; 15.4 g carbohydrate; 10.5 g sugar; 2.4 g
fiber; 27 mg sodium; 32 mg calcium; 1.3 mg iron; 0.1 mg vitamin C; 1
mcg beta-carotene; 0.2 mg vitamin E

Note: I used about ½ cup of non-dairy milk in a double batch to
soften the strong cocoa taste.

Chocolate Raspberry Mousse
From Physicians Committee for Responsible Medicine's 21-Day
Vegan Kick Start Program

Makes 4 ½ cup servings.

1 pound soft silken tofu
2 tablespoons cocoa powder
1/3 - ½ cup maple syrup (to taste)
1 teaspoon vanilla or raspberry extract (optional)
½ cup fresh raspberries

Place all ingredients in a blender and process until completely smooth.
Spoon into small bowls and chill well before serving.

210 calories/cup

Chocolate Cherry Nirvana Smoothie
From Food for Life 90-Day Journal by Physician's Committee for Responsible Medicine

Makes 4 servings.

2 cups frozen cherries
2 bananas
1 ½ cups chocolate non-dairy milk

Put all ingredients in blender and blend until smoothie consistency.

Per 0.25 of the recipe: 154 calories; 1.7 g fat; 0.3 g saturated fat; 10% of calories from fat; 0 mg cholesterol; 3.4 g protein; 33.8 g carbohydrate; 23.8 g sugar; 3.4 g fiber; 49 mg sodium; 127 mg calcium; 0.8 mg iron; 11.6 mg vitamin C; 44 mcg beta-carotene; 0.2 mg vitamin E

Nicer Krispie Squares
From Dreena Burton

Makes 16 squares.

½ cup macadamia nut butter (cashew butter will work too)
½ cup brown rice syrup
3 tablespoons unrefined sugar (can reduce or omit, to taste)
¼ teaspoon sea salt
¼ teaspoon agar powder (gelatin substitute available in health food
      stores)
1-1½ teaspoons pure vanilla extract
4 cups natural brown rice crisp cereal (available in most health food
      stores)

Line an 8"x8" pan with parchment paper. In a large saucepan on low-medium heat, combine macadamia nut butter, brown rice syrup, sugar, salt, agar powder, and vanilla. Stir continually as mixture heats until agar powder is fully dissolved (reduce heat if mixture starts bubbling). Remove from heat and stir in cereal, making sure to fully incorporate with nut butter mixture. Transfer mixture to pan and press evenly (use an edge of parchment paper to press without sticking). Refrigerate to cool completely, then cut into squares.

Quick Rice Pudding
From Physicians Committee for Responsible Medicine's Recipe of the Week

Makes 4 servings.

1½ cups plain or vanilla non-dairy milk
1 teaspoon cornstarch or arrowroot powder
2 cups cooked brown rice
¼ cup maple syrup
1/3 cup raisins
¼ teaspoon cinnamon
1 teaspoon vanilla extract
½ teaspoon almond extract

Put non-dairy milk into a medium saucepan and stir in cornstarch or arrowroot powder. Add rice, maple syrup, raisins, and cinnamon and bring to a simmer over medium heat.

Cook 3 minutes, then remove from heat and stir in vanilla and almond extracts.

Serve hot or cold.

Nutrition information per serving:

calories: 254; fat: 1.8 g; saturated fat: 0.3 g; calories from fat: 6.5%; cholesterol: 0 mg; protein: 5.7 g; carbohydrate: 53.9 g; sugar: 21.6 g; fiber: 1.8 g; sodium: 57 mg; calcium: 142 mg; iron: 2.4 mg; vitamin C: 0.6 mg; beta-carotene: 1 mcg; vitamin E: 1.3 mg

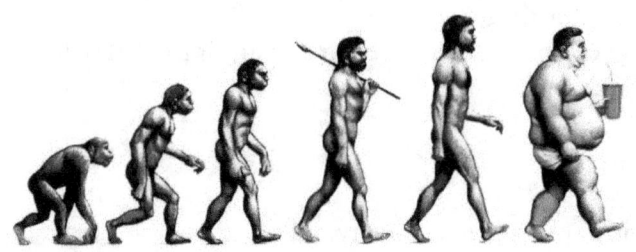

Additional Sources of Information

In addition to the information contained in this book, listed below are additional sources of information that are important enough that I encourage you to check them out:

My web site is packed with information and is continually being enhanced: http://www.traceyeakin.com.

Follow me on Pinterest: http://pinterest.com/traceyeakin/

Follow my blog: http://traceyeakin.wordpress.com/

Follow me on Twitter: @TraceyEakin1

Subscribe to my YouTube channel:
https://www.youtube.com/user/traceyeakin?feature=guide

Friend me on Facebook: Tracey Trombetta Eakin

Like and follow me on Facebook at Tracey Eakin: Plant-Based Nutrition Counselor.

Connect with me on LinkedIn: Tracey (Trombetta) Eakin

Follow my company on LinkedIn:
https://www.linkedin.com/company/3124931?trk=tyah&trkInfo=tarI d%3A1407678147855%2Ctas%3Atracey%20eakin%2C%20plant-ba%2Cidx%3A1-1-1

Follow this link to access articles that I have written: http://www.traceyeakin.com/articles.html

I am available for consultations and to speak to groups. I can be reached at traceyeakin@gmail.com or at 724.469.0693.

The sources of your information are as important as their message. They must be credible, trusted, their recommendations must be backed by scientifically credible research, and they shouldn't have a vested interest in what they are recommending. Listed below are my trusted sources for information. I go to them first when researching a question and look to them for additional trusted sources of information.

Michael Greger, MD

www.nutritionfacts.org

Dr. Greger scours the world's scholarly literature looking for credible research on nutrition's impact on our health. He summarizes his findings and provides practical advice for implementing positive changes in our lifestyle in brief videos that can be watched for free. These videos are enjoyed by both the medical profession and lay people. You can sign up to receive his videos every weekday via email.

If I could only recommend one source to follow, it would be Dr. Greger.

T. Colin Campbell, PhD

http://nutritionstudies.org/

Book: The China Study

Book: Whole

Dr. Campbell is Jacob Gould Schurman Professor Emeritus of Nutritional Biochemistry at Cornell University. He has received more than 70 grant-years of peer-reviewed research funding and authored more than 300 research papers. He led the most comprehensive research study on nutrition ever conducted, The China Study, which was the culmination of a 20-year partnership of Cornell University, Oxford University, and the Chinese Academy of Preventive Medicine. He is also the creator of Cornell University's Plant-Based Nutrition Program.

Caldwell B. Esselstyn, Jr., MD

www.heartattackproof.com

Book: Prevent and Reverse Heart Disease

Caldwell B. Esselstyn, Jr., received his B.A. from Yale University and his M.D. from Western Reserve University. He was trained as a surgeon at the Cleveland Clinic and at St. George's Hospital in London. Dr. Esselstyn has been associated with the Cleveland Clinic since 1968. His scientific publications number over 150. In 1995, he published his bench mark long-term nutritional research arresting and reversing coronary artery disease in severely ill patients. That same study was updated at 12 years and reviewed beyond 20 years in his book, Prevent and Reverse Heart Disease, making it one of the longest longitudinal studies of its type. Dr. Esselstyn presently directs the cardiovascular prevention and reversal program at The Cleveland Clinic Wellness Institute.

Neal D. Barnard, MD

http://pcrm.org/health/cancer-resources/

You can sign up to receive The Cancer Project's Food for Life Recipe of the Week email.

www.nealbarnard.org

www.pcrm.org

Book: The Cancer Survivor's Guide: Foods that help you Fight Back!

Book: Dr. Neal Barnard's Program for Reversing Diabetes: The Scientifically Proven System   for Reversing Diabetes Without Drugs

Book: Turn Off the Fat Genes: The Revolutionary Guide to Losing Weight

Book: A Physician's Slimming Guide

Book: Breaking the Food Seduction

Book: Power Foods for the Brain: An Effective 3-Step Plan to Protect Your Mind and   Strengthen Your Memory

Book: Foods That Fight Pain

Book: 21-Day Weight Loss Kickstart: Boost Metabolism, Lower Cholesterol, and Dramatically Improve your Health

John A. McDougall, MD

www.drmcdougall.com

Dr. McDougall's web site contains an extensive library of free and low-cost video presentations and audio versions of his Advanced Study Weekends.

He holds Advanced Study Weekends, runs a live-in program, and schedules periodic health adventures to Costa Rica and Hawaii.

Book: McDougall's Medicine: A Challenging Second Opinion

Book: Dr. McDougall's Digestive Tune-Up

Book: The Starch Solution

Book: The McDougall Program

Book: The McDougall Quick and Easy Cookbook: Over 300 Delicious Low-Fat Recipes You Can Prepare in Fifteen Minutes or Less

Matthew Lederman, MD

Conducted extensive research on the lack of sound, scientific evidence justifying artificial supplementation protocols that has led him to discourage any artificial supplementation with the exception of vitamin B_{12} and only under certain circumstances, vitamin D.

Book: Keep it Simple, Keep it Whole

Book: The Forks Over Knives Plan with Alona Pulde, MD

Documentary: Forks Over Knives

Michael Klaper, MD

True North Health Center

www.healthpromoting.com

Book: Vegan Nutrition: Pure and Simple

Book: Pregnancy, Children, and the Vegan Diet

Douglas J. Lisle, PhD

Book: The Pleasure Trap: Mastering the Hidden Force that Undermines Health & Happiness

Video: How to Lose Weight Without Losing Your Mind, https://www.youtube.com/watch?v=xAdqLB6bTuQ

Video: The Pleasure Trap, https://www.youtube.com/watch?v=TreRUEVxmT0

Video: The Willpower Paradox

Brendan Brazier

Brendan is a professional Ironman triathlete and is 100% plant-based.

www.vegasport.com

www.thriveforward.com

Book: Thrive Fitness: The Vegan-Based Training Program

Book: Thrive Foods: 200 Plant-Based Recipes for Peak Health

Robert Cheeke

www.veganbodybuilding.com

Book: Vegan Bodybuilding & Fitness

Jeff Novick, MS, RD, LD, LN

Other Cooking Demonstration Videos

www.FoodforLifeTV.org

Wonderful videos of cooking demonstrations including nutrition information and cooking tips from The Physician's Committee for Responsible Medicine

VegNews TV on www.youtube.com

www.youtube.com/user/vegnewstv?feature=results_main

Plant-Based Chefs

Susan Voisin, FatFree Vegan Kitchen

www.blog.fatfreevegan.com

Delicious recipes! This is my go to site!

Caroline Graettinger, PhD's Garden Dish

http://www.gardendish.com/Caroline makes planning, shopping, and cooking plant-based easy! Her Monthly Dish provides 20 seasonally-selected recipes each month, along with the nutrition information for each recipe. You have the ability to automatically generate shopping lists based on which recipe(s) you want to cook, and you have access to a growing database of delicious meal ideas.

Dreena Burton's Plant Powered Kitchen

http://plantpoweredkitchen.com/

Kathy Patalsky

http://kblog.lunchboxbunch.com/

More great recipes!

Chef AJ

http://chefajonline.com/

Book: Unprocessed

Patty Knutson

A personal chef in Reno, Nevada that has a very informative web site that helps you to learn how to make delicious vegan meals with or without recipes

www.vegancoach.com

Plant-Based Dining Guide

www.VeganPittsburgh.com

To locate vegan restaurants in the Pittsburgh area.

www.happycow.net

To locate vegan and vegetarian-friendly restaurants around the world.

Other Credible Sources of Medical Information

The Cochrane Collaboration

http://www.cochrane.org/

The Cochrane Collaboration is one of the highest authorities in medical research.

Informed Medical Decisions Foundation

http://informedmedicaldecisions.org/what-is-shared-decision-making/

Provides patients and their families with unbiased, evidenced-based information about the available options and possible outcomes so that the patient is better equipped to make an informed medical decision that is aligned with their preferences.

Number Needed to Treat

www.thennt.com

A physician-maintained web site that utilizes a framework and rating system that they developed to evaluate therapies based on their *patient-important* benefits and harms as well as a system to evaluate diagnostics by patient sign, symptom, lab test, or study. They use only the highest quality, evidenced-based studies (frequently, but not always Cochrane reviews) and they accept no outside funding or advertisements.

Dartmouth Atlas of Health Care

http://www.dartmouthatlas.org/

Enables you to determine if your community has higher rates of different types of surgery than the national norm. It will not necessarily help you to make a medical decision that is right for you, but can provide you with insight that the treatment your doctor recommends may not depend entirely on you and your medical condition, but also on how doctors in your community practice medicine.

HealthNewsReview.org

Provides independent, expert reviews of news stories.

IndUShealth

http://www.indushealth.com/intro_video.aspx

Founded by a former U.S. hospital CEO to help patients evaluate their global medical options.

Environmental Working Group

www.ewg.org

For information on pesticides, herbicides, and other chemicals. Creators of the Dirty Dozen (pesticide laden produce to buy organic if at all possible) and the Clean 15 (produce that contains lower levels of pesticides that can be purchased conventionally grown if need be).

Additional Informative Books

Whitewash: The Disturbing Truth About Cow's Milk and Your Health by Joseph Keon and John Robbins (former heir to the Baskin-Robbins empire who walked away from it due to the dangers of dairy)

The End of Overeating: Taking Control of the Insatiable American Appetite by David A. Kessler, MD

This book is helpful in trying to understand the impact that food layered and loaded with added fat, sugar, and salt can have on our brain chemistry and how the food industry exploits this to their advantage, but I would not recommend the book's food-specific recommendations as they contradict what sound, scientific studies demonstrate as the optimal way to nourish ourselves.

The Fluoride Deception by Christopher Bryson

Overdiagnosed: Making People Sick in the Pursuit of Health by Drs. H. Gilbert Welch, Lisa M.   Schwartz, and Steven Woloshin

The Treatment Trap: How the Overuse of Medical Care is Wrecking Your Health and What You Can Do to Prevent It by Rosemary Gibson and Janardan Prasad Singh

The Engine 2 Diet by Rip Esselstyn

Forks Over Knives: The Plant-Based Way to Health

Skinny Bitch by Rory Freedman and Kim Barnouin (a very informative book but delivered using very vulgar language)

Skinny Bitch in the Kitch by Rory Freedman and Kim Barnouin (great recipes but again, very vulgar language)

Vegan for Life: Everything You Need to Know to be Healthy and Fit on a Plant-Based Diet by Jack Norris, RD and Virginia Messina, MPH, RD

Overcoming Multiple Sclerosis: An Evidenced-Based Guide to Recovery by Professor George Jelinek

Unraveling the Mystery of Autism and Pervasive Development Disorder, A Mother's Story of Research and Recovery by Karyn Seroussi

Finding Ultra: Rejecting Middle Age, Becoming One of the World's Fittest Men, and Finding Myself by Rich Roll

Superbug: The Fatal Menace of MRSA by Maryn McKenna

Let It Rot! The Gardener's Guide to Composting by Stu Campbell

Additional Informative DVDs

Forks Over Knives

Cowspiracy

PlantPure Nation (not yet released on DVD)

Super Size Me starring Morgan Spurlock

Forks Over Knives Presents The Engine 2 Kitchen Rescue with Rip Esselstyn

From Oil to Nuts: The Essential Facts of Fats, Oils, and Nuts by Jeff Novick, MS, RD, LD, LN

Nuts and Health: What the Science Really Says by Jeff Novick, MS, RD, LD, LN

Chow Down

Vegucated

About the Author

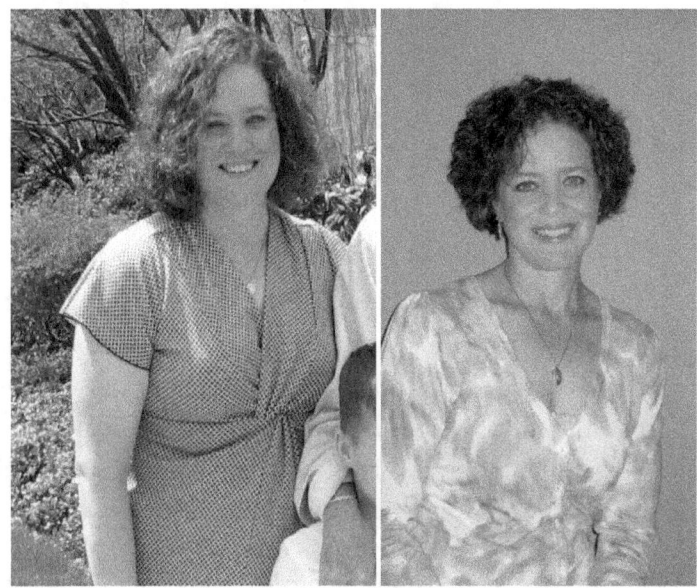

Before (left picture) and After (right picture) Adopting a Plant-Based Lifestyle

My Background

With an undergraduate and graduate degree in finance and 13 years of experience in the corporate finance world, I chose to switch careers in order to share what I've learned about how food choices can affect our health and likelihood of disease.

I completed *the only collegiate program in the country* focused on the medical benefits of a plant-based lifestyle from Cornell University. The curriculum is grounded in the most comprehensive studies of nutrition conducted to-date. I am also certified by John McDougall, MD, one of the most respected medical doctors in the field of plant-based nutrition, to teach his program, The Starch Solution. I am a

Board Certified Holistic Health Practitioner by the American Association of Drugless Practitioners.

In 2013-2014, I was asked to be the Technical Editor of Plant-Based Diet for Dummies for John Wiley & Sons Publishing. The purpose of my technical review was to ensure the accuracy and completeness of the information presented in the book.

In 2014, I partnered with Cynthia West, MD to create Lifestyle WoR$_x$. Lifestyle WoR$_x$ is an evidenced-based lifestyle improvement program. It is designed to help participants to improve their health and how they feel by adopting a multi-faceted approach to wellness. The cornerstone of the program is the pursuit of dietary excellence, but also incorporates increasing activity levels into an already busy schedule, and more effectively managing stress.

Lifestyle WoR$_x$'s creative programming covers a wide range of chronic, degenerative diseases such as vascular disease (including heart disease and stroke), type II diabetes, overweight/obesity, gastrointestinal disorders, autoimmune conditions, cancer, and osteoporosis that can be prevented, arrested, reversed, or more effectively battled with judicious lifestyle choices. Lifestyle WoR$_x$ is now credentialed with the following insurance carriers: Highmark, UPMC, Coventry/HealthAmerica/Aetna, Cigna, United Healthcare, and Medicare.

This lifestyle choice has made a significant difference in my health. I was able to lose over 50 pounds and maintain the weight loss. I resolved an autoimmune condition known as idiopathic thrombocytopenic purpura or ITP. My body was attacking and destroying my platelets. I could have faced the removal of my spleen or platelet transfusions. My total cholesterol plummeted from 197 to 132 without medication. According to Dr. Esselstyn, I am now heart attack proof. I just don't have enough saturated fat and cholesterol in my body to cause a cardiac event. My left knee was osteoarthritic. I had it reconstructed after a gymnastics accident and have had a total of five surgeries as doctors attempted to delay a total knee replacement until I was old enough to have one. As of the time of this writing, I am almost three years overdue for my next surgery. My arthritic pain melted away when I gave up dairy and as of now, I have no intention of having my knee replaced. A low-fat, plant-based lifestyle made a dramatic difference in my life.

My Approach

I present a new paradigm for nutrition, one which is based on sound, evidenced-based research, to enable people not only to prevent, reverse, or battle chronic, degenerative disease, but also to achieve optimal health through dietary excellence.

I meet with people individually or in groups to introduce them to the enormous benefits of a plant-based lifestyle and to show them that it is easier to adopt than most people think.

Research indicates that it takes approximately three weeks to change a habit and our taste buds. I help interested clients "test drive" this new way of living for three weeks and then if clients want to continue feeling fabulous and full of energy, I assist them with a more permanent transition.

I also founded Lifestyle WoR$_x$ with Cynthia West, MD. Lifestyle WoR$_x$ helps participants to reclaim their health by showing them how to incorporate healthy eating, increased activity, and stress management habits into their busy lives. This program accepts most insurance plans.

Are You Struggling with a Chronic Condition?

Your food choices can significantly impact your ability to prevent, resolve, or battle a chronic condition. Are you willing to give yourself just 3 weeks to test drive a low-cost, side effect-free alternative to a lifetime of repeated surgeries, drugs, and side effects?

Contact Me

I help people to achieve their wellness goals by providing them with the tools that they need to gain control over their health. If you would like individualized assistance with your weight, with a chronic, degenerative disease, with other health and wellness aspirations, or if you would like me to speak to a group, please email me at traceyeakin@gmail.com or give me a call at 724.469.0693 to arrange a time.

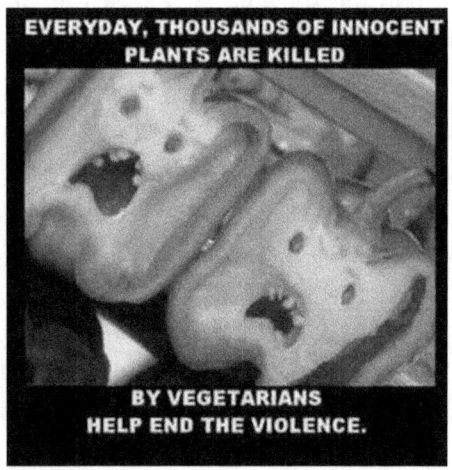

www.ingramcontent.com/pod-product-compliance
Lightning Source LLC
Chambersburg PA
CBHW071031290526
45795CB00004B/1173